T0298688

"This book is an important contribution to the sociological study of pandemics and life-saving bodily donations as well as medical uncertainty and even human uncertainty more generally. It also has the distinctive merit of bringing new questions and new theoretical insights to research on liminality, gifts, and the relation between them. This book convincingly highlights processual, time-related, and intertwined dynamics of illness, liminality, and gifts, which we can only hope will inspire similar explorations of various types of life-saving donations in other national contexts and possibly enrich research on gift-giving in other spheres of social life."

Ilana F. Silber, *Professor of Anthropology and Sociology at Bar-Ilan University, Israel; Coeditor-in-chief of the journal* MAUSS International

"This book offers an incredible opportunity to examine classical sociological theory in the context of the pandemic. It provides invaluable insights for those who recognize the potential of future global-scale infectious diseases. It is also a perfect example of how qualitative research can significantly enhance our understanding of the human experience during the interruption of everyday life caused by COVID-19. The authors successfully demonstrate the immense power of semantic theory construction through cultural interpretation, contextualization, and capturing multiple dimensions of lived experience, ultimately revealing the dynamic and emergent nature of social reality. With its insightful analysis and practical advice, readers will be empowered to take control of their lives and make a positive impact on the world."

Jaeyeol Yee, *Professor of Sociology at Seoul National University, S. Korea*

A Sociological Perspective on Blood Plasma Donation During the Pandemic

Shim and Baek examine the evolving existential meanings of gift-making by interviewing donors of convalescent blood plasma during the COVID-19 pandemic.

The book reveals what plasma donation means for their efforts to reassemble their lives from being liminal moments to livable experiences, through interviews with convalescent donors in South Korea. It shows it is the very multiplex meanings of plasma donations that enabled people to effectively maneuver through the challenging liminality in life during COVID-19, by expanding the existing literature on gifts and donations that highlights the rich, complex meanings of the body parts donated. It presents a vivid dialogue between liminality and gift-making from varied narratives.

A vital read for scholars, students of sociology, anthropology, and public health and those interested in how subjects reconstitute their agency amid uncertainty inside and outside the pandemic, so that we appreciate the voices of donors and learn from the lived experiences of those in this book.

Jae-Mahn Shim is Professor of Sociology at Korea University.

Seung-Hyun Baek is a Chief of the Resource Mobilization & Public Relations Center at the Korean National Commission for UNESCO.

Routledge Advances in Sociology

For more information about this series, please visit: https://www.routledge.com/Routledge-Advances-in-Sociology/book-series/SE0511

A Sociological Perspective on Blood Plasma Donation During the Pandemic

Convalescent Gifts and Liminality

Jae-Mahn Shim and
Seung-Hyun Baek

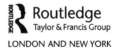

LONDON AND NEW YORK

First published 2025
by Routledge
4 Park Square, Milton Park, Abingdon, Oxon OX14 4RN

and by Routledge
605 Third Avenue, New York, NY 10158

Routledge is an imprint of the Taylor & Francis Group, an informa business

British Library Cataloguing-in-Publication Data
A catalogue record for this book is available from the British Library

Library of Congress Cataloging-in-Publication Data
Names: Shim, Jae-Mahn, author. | Baek, Seung-Hyun, author.
Title: A sociological perspective on blood plasma donation during the
pandemic : convalescent gifts and liminality / Jae-Mahn Shim,
Seung-Hyun Baek.
Description: Abingdon, Oxon ; New York, NY : Routledge, 2025. |
Series: Routledge advances in sociology | Includes bibliographical
references and index.
Identifiers: LCCN 2024026453 (print) | LCCN 2024026454 (ebook) |
ISBN 9781032797564 (hardback) | ISBN 9781032797595 (paperback) |
ISBN 9781003493723 (ebook)
Subjects: LCSH: Plasma exchange (Therapeutics)--Social aspects--Korea
(South) | Blood donors--Korea (South)--Psychology. |
Blood donors--Korea (South)--Social conditions. | COVID-19 Pandemic,
2020---Korea (South)--Influence. | COVID-19 Pandemic, 2020---Social
aspects--Korea (South)
Classification: LCC RM175 .S55 2025 (print) |
LCC RM175 (ebook) | DDC 615.3/9--dc23/eng/20240613
LC record available at https://lccn.loc.gov/2024026453
LC ebook record available at https://lccn.loc.gov/2024026454

ISBN: 978-1-032-79756-4 (hbk)
ISBN: 978-1-032-79759-5 (pbk)
ISBN: 978-1-003-49372-3 (ebk)

DOI: 10.4324/9781003493723

Typeset in Galliard
by KnowledgeWorks Global Ltd.

For Sophia, Eunjung, and many gift-makers

Contents

Acknowledgments

The authors deliver special thanks to all the donors interviewed in the book. This work was supported by the Ministry of Education of the Republic of Korea and the National Research Foundation of Korea (NRF-2020S1A5A2A01043365).

Introduction

Liminality

Uncertainties that people manage to live through during the coronavirus disease-2019 (COVID-19) pandemic concern sociology (Kosar & Kasapoglu, 2021; Rebughini, 2021; Ward, 2020; Ward et al., 2022; Zinn, 2021). Suspense, fear, and doubts have been commonplace regarding whether one is already or really infected; whether one has recovered or is ever recoverable from the infection in meaningful ways – e.g., discourses of "long" COVID; whether one is more or less susceptible to contracting the viruses; whether the face-mask and vaccines salvage people from the infection; when this pandemic will end and when it will resurge; whether one can get back to "normal" years; how the future – i.e., "the new normal" – may and should look; whether one heads back to the same, old social systems and individual identities; whether one should willingly or forcibly dream of new orders and individualities; and, if so, to what extent. In brief, suspense, suspicion, and doubts surrounding the COVID-19 uncertainties are multivocal. They span medical, economic, political, social, and cultural areas. In each area, they are not related only to destructive but also (re-)generative processes and consequences that the viruses and people's response to them co-produce.

How social actors deal with uncertainties is one of the major topics among medical sociological studies on health experiences (Lupton, 1995; Mackintosh & Armstrong, 2020; Shim, 2022; Timmermans & Buchbinder, 2010). Medical sociology has long been attentive to uncertainties and social contestations that are necessary for defining what illness, treatment, recovery, or health means (Brown, 1995; Conrad, 2005; Timmermans & Haas, 2008). In the general sociological perspective, these medical sociological categories are typical examples of the taken-for-granted categories and objectivities that are actually experienced among people as blurry boundaries (Lamont & Molnár, 2002; Star & Griesemer, 1989) or negotiable knowledge (Berger & Luckmann, 1991 [1967]) that are not fixed but dynamically unfolding in process. Similar

DOI: 10.4324/9781003493723-1

processual experiences are widespread, and uncertainties prevail in almost all aspects of social life. Accordingly, this book turns to one of the general sociological imaginations that address uncertainties as the focal topic, the sociology of liminality (Turner, 1967, 1982, 1985a, 1991 [1969]; van Gennep, 1960 [1909]). This book finds the multifold meanings of liminality in the literature to be especially relevant to understanding life experiences during the current pandemic.

Surrounded by viruses, individuals suddenly turn liminal, and they respond to liminality in various ways that produce different implications for their lives. When infected with mysterious, "emerging" viruses (Jerolmack, 2013; Jones et al., 2008), individuals are placed outside the conventional socio-cultural status categories, such as the ill and the healthy. They are not healthy anymore because they are found positive in the disputable infection tests; they are not ill in any definitive sense either because valid treatments, reliable prognoses, or preventive measures are not firmly in place yet for emerging infectious diseases. In this sense, the infected remain both healthy and ill; they are neither healthy nor ill; alas, they are *both* and *neither* in the Turnerian sense (Turner, 1967). This seemingly blurry situation applies no less to people who have never been infected. Although not infected, individuals are always at risk of infection. They are not sanguine or healthy; they are not downcast or ill either; they are neither healthy nor ill; they are both healthy and ill; yes, they are both and neither. Meanwhile, all these people are put on the margin and threshold of social relations – due to quarantine and social distancing – within the family, at school, and at work for days, weeks, months, and even years because they are a risk to others or at risk of being infected. Living through liminality becomes a critical concern not only for people infected with the viruses but also for those who are at risk of infection.

One way to comprehend this situation lies in the sociology of liminality pioneered by Arnold van Gennep and generalized by Victor Turner. The literature posits that liminal experiences are essential and fundamental to human existence. First, the classics suggest that people cannot help but encounter unconventional, monstrous, and scandalous events at various points in life where they are placed outside the known socio-cultural categories and instead put on the margins, limens, thresholds, and interstices of established categories. Second, once they encounter liminality, individuals manage to live through it in various ways. Third, the literature implies that different ways to live through liminality lead to varying consequences for individual and collective lives. This study conceptualizes all these three aspects as *the ways of liminality*.

Different ways of liminality – how people are put into liminality, how they respond to it, and what consequences liminality brings to people depending on how they respond to it – have been sporadically implied in the literature on several occasions. According to van Gennep's famous three-stage model (van Gennep, 1960 [1909]), people lead into (i.e., preliminal separation), stay with (i.e., liminality), and get out of liminality (i.e., reintegration or incorporation). In another formulation, some individuals choose to be led into liminality (e.g., performance arts and religious pilgrimage) (Turner, 1985b; Turner & Turner, 1978), while others are involuntarily forced into it (e.g., subjects in most rituals of passage) (Turner, 1967; van Gennep, 1960 [1909]). The former voluntary liminality is likely what individuals want to stay with, while the latter forced liminality is what individuals want to get out of in due time. In a third formulation, some people experience liminality only transiently, while others live with it for a long time or permanently (Turner, 1967, 1991 [1969]; van Gennep, 1960 [1909]), being exposed to various consequences. In a fourth formulation, some people experience liminality as a source of generative power that reinvigorates and reinvents their life, while others experience it as a destructive power that hampers and derails routine life (Turner, 1985b, 1991 [1969]; Turner & Turner, 1978).

While being driven home by the literature to the sociological insight that liminality is a necessary part of human existence as a social and biosocial being, this study remains puzzled by a lack of further theorization on the seemingly divergent ways in which individuals turn into, respond to, and get affected by liminality. Regarding the classics, it is not sufficient to simply suggest that liminal experiences are "building blocks" of culture for human existence (Turner, 1967, p. 110) without elaborating on specific ways in which building blocks materialize themselves. Neither is sufficient to adumbrate that some people (opt to) lead into and stay with liminality, anticipating positive consequences, while others (try to) get away from it, avoiding adverse effects. Given the essentiality of liminality for human existence, liminality is what all individuals learn experientially to live through rather than what they intend to attain or avoid as they wish. The latter purposeful aspect constitutes only a part of the former experiential process. It is one thing to recognize liminality as central to human existence; it is another to complicate and enrich it in its varying modes and ways in practice. Therefore, many expect subsequent studies to elaborate on the various manners, ways, and modes in which individuals learn to live through liminality (Horvath et al., 2015, p. 232; Lamond & Moss, 2020; Mountz, 2011; O'Reilly, 2018, p. 839).

Subsequent studies have not fully met the expectations. Most studies have failed to comprehend all three underlying concerns of the classics in a coherent way: that is, the undeniable presence of life turning liminal at times; various efforts to live through liminality; and the rich consequences of these efforts. Most often, studies focus on delivering the first concern only and demonstrate the conceptual validity of liminality to different empirical contexts such as international migration (Aguilar, 2018 [1999]; Menjívar, 2006), transnational asylum-seeking

(Ghorashi et al., 2017; O'Reilly, 2018), international relations/wars (Atanasova, 2019; Malksoo, 2015), emergent work/labor (Czarniawska & Mazza, 2003; Kim et al., 2020), human development (Joseph et al., 2019; Silver, 1996; Suárez-Orozco et al., 2011), trans-sexuality (Wilson, 2002; Wimark, 2021), illness/health experiences via health-monitoring technologies (Forss et al., 2004; Scott et al., 2005), organ transplants (Cormier et al., 2017; Wiltshire et al., 2020), end-of-life care (Jordan et al., 2015; MacArtney et al., 2017), and bereavement (Kim, 2021).

Regarding a handful of studies that address the second concern (Cormier et al., 2017; Czarniawska & Mazza, 2003; Ekins & King, 1999; Wilson, 2002), it is regrettable to witness that these studies lack comparing the ways of living liminality that they find with the ways that are already insinuated in the classics. Due to this neglect, a promising conceptual dialogue with the classics (Szakolczai, 2017) implying that liminality can be lived with the help of another instance of liminality – "the heart" – or a firm category – "the mind" – has been lost in the literature. Theoretical negligence is costly on another front. The studies do not attempt to investigate further what consequences each of these different ways may produce at the individual and collective levels – i.e., how their lives are reconstituted – which are, according to the classics, the most crucial concerns for liminal subjects and to which the classics do not have rich answers yet. Likewise, studies that explicitly or implicitly examine the third concern – consequences of liminal experiences – fall short of advancing the classics' suggestion that different ways of living liminality may lead to different consequences by not relating their findings on the consequences to the varying ways to respond to liminality (Menjívar, 2006; Pozzo & Ghorashi, 2021; Suárez-Orozco et al., 2011; Wiltshire et al., 2020).

This book posits that the unanswered central problematic in the classics can be adequately addressed by an inquiry to apprehend how individuals live *through* liminality. This study proposes a long-waited *holistic* understanding of liminal experiences that covers all three aspects of the ways of liminality and, subsequently, a proper account of the lived experiences during the pandemic. To this end, it listens to the voices of some survivors of COVID-19.

Convalescent Plasma Donations

While there are various groups of infected individuals across the world, this study focuses on South Koreans who have survived the infection and *bothered to give* for free their blood plasma – which is rich with natural antibodies against the viruses – to medical institutions for immediate treatment of the infected others in critical conditions or for developing manufactured remedies targeted at the drug market. While the scientific foundation for survivors' plasma-based therapies is ever in the making

(Kupferschmidt, 2020) and is only recently qualified through randomized controlled trials (Rubin, 2022; Thomas & Weiland, 2021), this study is intrigued by those donating survivors and the uncommon efforts they make for donation.

The survivors have had to go through several discouraging obstacles to make their donation finally, such as the moralized blaming – for their being infected earlier than others and putting others at increased risks of infection – and distancing toward the infected, which have been commonplace during the early period, and the geographical remoteness and scarcity of donation-accepting medical facilities in the middle of national lockdown – only four medical centers throughout Korea during the early months of the pandemic. The fact that less than 10% of all COVID-19-surviving Koreans have donated or pledged to donate their plasma shows that the donation is anything but natural. This Korean context is not atypical compared to what is uncovered by a brief survey of how other countries have implemented convalescent plasma therapy and donations during these years.

Convalescent plasma therapy has recurred in the medical history. It is "a treatment more than a century old that has gone in and out of fashion: in when infectious disease outbreaks occurred and then out when treatments and vaccines that could be mass-produced were developed to contain them. Taken from healthy people who have recovered from the infectious disease of interest, antibody-rich convalescent plasma is thought to give recipients' immune systems a running start" (Rubin, 2020, p. 2114). The latest recommendation about plasma therapy among the world health community as of 2022 is that it is limitedly efficacious for early stage infections, old-aged patients, and those with weak immune systems (Rubin, 2022).

Within these medical scientific limits, countless efforts have been made to procure COVID-19 survivors' plasma worldwide during the early months of the pandemic, with no vaccines or valid treatment remedies available. Like in Korea, plasma is collected to treat infected people in critical conditions or develop plasma-based marketable cures in clinical trials. An international survey identifies 64 centers in 22 countries conducting clinical trials on plasma therapy since the outbreak until May 2020 (Murphy et al., 2020). The procurement predominantly takes forms of voluntary donation, reflecting the World Health Organization's (WHO) recommendation that plasma be collected from voluntary, unpaid donors. Implementations vary in detail regarding this "non-renumerated donation" among countries and organizations within a country. Most contexts allow in-kind gifts in return for donations, such as refreshments, gift certificates, and free medical check-ups to donors, while some countries – Austria, the Czech Republic, Germany, the United States, etc. – feature monetary remuneration equivalent to transportation costs or higher (Pant et al., 2021).

Several adversities have beleaguered plasma procurement based on donors' volunteerism. Most recruitment efforts are made through the public media, advertising procurement programs, and facilities without guaranteed turnouts. Yet reaching out to potential donors via medical staff's phone calls to those recovered is fraught with privacy infringement issues (Appiah, 2020; Bloch et al., 2020). In addition, potential donors have to bear medical, psychological, and social burdens to make donations ultimately. As it is reported that 16–40% of donated convalescent plasma do not have antibodies (Wendel et al., 2021), many donation drives require a pre-donation medical test for health conditions and the minimum levels of antibodies in plasma often at a few selected medical facilities during the early period of the pandemic (Li et al., 2020; Terada et al., 2021; Wade et al., 2021), which takes additional commitment from potential donors. On a psychological front, plasma procurement has caused among potential donors anxiety and fear not only about the unfamiliar, uncomfortable procurement procedure – needles and plasmapheresis – but also about getting sick again after their plasma is drawn out of their bodies (Crowder et al., 2023; Masser et al., 2021; Roberts et al., 2020). Amid a local or national lockdown, visiting a facility with the fear of reinfection has made it more challenging to participate in plasma donations (Maheshwari et al., 2022).

Nonetheless, there are pockets of people in different countries who seem eager to donate plasma against the adversities, like a donor who traveled a long distance by bicycle during the lockdown to a donation facility several times a week (Harmon, 2020). A survey of donors in the United States during the first five months of plasma donation – April to September 2020 – finds that 41% of plasma donors have never donated blood before, and 30% are lapsed donors who have taken at least two years since their last blood donation (Crowder et al., 2023). Another study finds that over half of the 59,000 volunteers who registered for convalescent plasma donation have never donated blood before (Lasky et al., 2021). Yet these highly motivated donors are not a majority among those who have recovered from the infection. An April report in 2021 finds that there are over 722,000 units of plasma supplied across the United States (Thomas & Weiland, 2021), which is about 2% of the cumulative infection cases in the country. In an early effort for plasma procurement in Shanghai in February 2020, only 14 out of the 124 recovered people showed the intention to donate (Mu, 2020; Yan, 2020). As of January 2021, China's National Health Commission pronounced over 4,700 donations (Huaxia, 2021), less than 5% of the total confirmed infection cases nationwide. In most countries – China, the United States, Italy, Japan, the United Kingdom, and South Korea – plasma donations are unusual gifts.

Gifts

One of Mauss's questions (Mauss, 1990 [1925]) is relevant to the current inquiry on the lived experiences of COVID-19 among plasma donors. While this study asks why survivors bother to give their blood plasma for free despite various adversities, Mauss asks why people feel obliged to give material goods – as well as "banquets, rituals, military services, women, children, dances, festivals, and fairs" (ibid., p. 5) – to others for free. Despite the spatial and temporal distance, there is an unmistakable resonance between the archaic societies in the classic and the world in the current pandemic. Indeed, Mauss proposes his theory of gift society as a general sociological perspective applicable to contemporary social practices. To that extent, Mauss provides a relevant, if not sufficient, answer to the current inquiry.

Let's begin with the empirical surprise about plasma donors. Why do the COVID-19 survivors bother to donate their plasma for free despite difficulties? The most common and immediate explanation is that people donate on account of the political (e.g., government campaigns), economic (e.g., drug companies' investments), and professional-scientific (e.g., practicing and research doctors' appeals) mobilization of donors' altruism under the current system of gift-making and donation. While it sounds simple and obvious, this answer is not self-sufficient and begets more questions. Speaking of the mobilization part, what are the mobilizations like? What ideas and materials do those mobilizers tap into? How do potential donors respond to them in their acts and voices? Do the mobilizers and potential donors coalesce or conflict with each other? Regarding altruism, what is altruism? Is altruism opposite to self-interest, inclusive of it, or included in it? What is self-interest vis-à-vis altruism? With regard to the given system of gift-making, what is the gift system like? Is it different from the market exchange system? How are the two related to each other? What is a market economy? What is a gift economy?

After all, one of the most fundamental inquiries is to delve into what a gift, giving, or donation is – otherwise, what commodity or market is. *The Gift* by Marcel Mauss (Mauss, 1990 [1925]) stands at this juncture, raising a series of fundamental questions. Why do people bother to give to others for free? How is this oxymoron – a free obligation or obliged freedom – possible? What does it reveal? In posing these questions, Mauss does not overlook the significance of self-interest and selfish individuals. He does not trivialize the importance of altruism, either. Instead, he acknowledges self-interest and altruism at once, ingeniously by not pitting them against each other but relating them while distinguishing them. In his treatment, they are not only distinct and correlative but also consubstantial; they are not only interdependent but also interpenetrative.

In giving material goods and services for free to an alter, Mauss begins to elaborate in the book, the ego lives up to the imperative of the ego's survival and existence. By making an alter live and depend on the ego's provision of material goods, the ego enables the alter's material existence and simultaneously secures a foundation of the ego's material existence in an interdependent world – as long as the alter lives whom the ego depends on, the ego increases its chance. In this world, self-interest resides not only in securing the self – the acting self (Coleman, 1990) – but also in sustaining others – the object self. In addition, gift-giving generates control power over the alter and promotes the chances for the ego's existence. This control power is multifold. It is ethical and moral power in the sense that the alter who receives material goods from the ego feels indebted or inferior to the ego, depending on the context, so that the alter is put under moral pressure to reciprocate with no less than what the alter initially receives. Impending and fulfilled reciprocation, such as social honor, reputation, and material returns, promises the ego's existence. The control power is also spiritual as it is believed that material goods from the ego involve not only the utilitarian value but the spiritual part – "hau" – of the giving ego. Once an alter receives a good, the alter also receives the hau of the ego that, if not returned back to the ego, stays and controls the alter as the ego wishes. This movement of hau and its control power assist the ego's existence. Mauss generalizes the presence of the spiritual side to a gift exchange by referring to the typical material offerings that people make to deities. When people (attempt to) make peace and reconcile with supernatural powers via offerings and sacrifices, they confess that spirituality inhabits material goods. Offerings are moments that reveal the underlying materiality–spirituality unity. In sum, people give goods for free to others for the sake of others' material survival and the ego's multifarious control power over others, which all contribute to the ego's survival and existence. In this formalization, self-interest and altruism are correlative and consubstantial; not only two related different things but also the same two things.

Consubstantiality, or the same two things like the self-interest–altruism complex and, in an extension, the same multiple things like a gift as the material–moral–spiritual complex, are often difficult to appreciate fully. A telling example is Pierre Bourdieu. He adopts the Weberian multidimensional worldview that should be conducive to appreciating consubstantiality. However, he still finds consubstantiality in a gift to be challenging. This challenge likely stems from his simultaneous embrace of the Marxist unidimensional, reductionist worldview that cannot but be tempted toward the primacy of one dimension over the others – especially the economic dimension. In his latest discussion of gifts (Bourdieu, 2000, pp. 188–202), his attempted appreciation of consubstantiality in a gift is clearly hampered by his recurring disposition toward the unequal, reductionist treatment of calculability vis-à-vis generosity despite his Weberian admission of their distinctiveness. In "The twofold truth of the gift," Bourdieu reasons that people who give and take gifts are caught between two different logics – altruistic generosity and self-interested calculation. Mauss sees these people not as being caught up by the two different logics but simply living on them. Mauss does not necessarily see such a gift exchange as a problem but as a window that reveals the multivocal nature of human action. In contrast, Bourdieu ponders on it as a problem that adumbrates one fundamental logic of action with other confusing, deceptive logic. In Bourdieu's perspective, people give and take a gift under the "self-deception" and "hypocrisy" of free generosity which masks the underlying logic of calculation. This lingering reductionism is revealed in Bourdieu in the opposite direction, as well. When a person takes a gift as calculation, that is in fact out of generosity and not calculation, the person is said to be deceived, not seeing the true nature of the gift, or generosity (for a comprehensive elaboration of Bourdieu's achievements and limitations in dealing with the gift across his several works culminating in the "The Twofold Truth of the Gift," see Silber, 2009). Mauss does not necessarily call such a gift exchange a problem situation in which one should tell apart true and false intentions but establishes it as the essence of reality in which two different logics coexist in a single exchange – the same two things. In context, one or the other logic may dominate.

This tension between Bourdieu's reductionism and Mauss's holism continues in another form in their treatments of time in gift relations. Mauss implies that the time that a person takes making a return gift generates multivocality of the return – i.e., multiple meanings that the return signifies – and this multivocality makes the return de facto a gift that carries not a single but plural meanings. Time enriches a return gift with multiple meanings, Mauss implies. However, Bourdieu treats such time only as a kind of interruption that makes the return look like not a return – i.e., a continuous happening that succeeds the preceding gift taken and an act of calculation – but a "discontinuous" happening and an act of generosity. Bourdieu suggests that time disguises a return gift with confusing meanings. Bourdieu reveals unidimensional reductionism in stressing either a calculating act of returning or a generous act of newly initiating a discontinued gift. In contrast, Mauss always begins the inquiry with multidimensional holism, overlooking both calculation and generosity. In sum, while Bourdieu describes duality or consubstantiality only as self-deception and hypocrisy, Mauss takes it as it is and even exaggerates it as a totality – a total social fact – that is, nonetheless, open to a full range of further developments involving not only hypocrisy and deception but many other possibilities like partiality as well as totality, singularity as well as plurality.

It is a relatively trivial task to read correlativity and consubstantiality from Mauss. What is more consequential is the implication that this Maussian formalization brings forth with regard to the nature of individual survival and existence, that is, the way of a human being and the self (Mauss, 1973 [1934]; Mauss, 1985 [1938]). First, human existence is relational as well as personal, and social as well as individual. That is why individual self-interests result in and coexist with collective goods in gift relations. Second, gift relations reveal that individual existence is not only material but moral and spiritual; not only spiritual but material. Since existence extends as far as the spiritual realm – the allegedly remotest possible from the material realm, it is multivocal, multivalent, and multidimensional, including all the known and yet-to-be-known realms of life that emerge between the two extremes, like politics, aesthetics, and more. On this basis, Mauss concludes that people feel obliged to give gifts to others because they live and exist as *total social services* or *totality*. In other words, people perform and govern themselves as total services, not only reflected in but also reconstituted by gifts. Regarding plasma donations during the pandemic, likewise, Mauss would answer that donors feel obliged toward free donations because they live and exist as total social services and total human beings who govern themselves both in person and in relations and, subsequently, in all possible realms of life, such as religion, economy, politics, intimacy, and the like (for an explication of how the notion of a total human being develops through the early 1920s and culminates in *The Gift*, see Garces & Jones, 2009 arguing even that Mauss's totalizing tendency does not stop at an individual or national level but extends to the international level, embracing the notion of globalization and globality; for an extended discussion of how a total social fact relates to the notion of a total human being, see Gofman, 1998).

If true indeed, one needs to complicate how this allegedly structuralist proposition of totality – in the sense that Mauss characterizes totality not only with "a very large number of institutions" but "the totality of society and its institutions" (Mauss, 1990 [1925], p. 78) – plays out as experiential life journeys among the COVID-19 survivors. This is what Mauss invites, who is believed to be as phenomenological and subjective as structuralist and objective in addressing the notion of totality (Garces & Jones, 2009; Gofman, 1998; Silber, 2009). What is this totality interest or gift interest like during the pandemic? What is so unique to the pandemic in which people bother donating plasma? Answering these questions, in turn, expands the Maussian thesis of totality by addressing the following questions that Mauss and subsequent studies – advocates and critics alike – have not examined sufficiently: do people bother to give anytime anywhere? Do people seek to live total anytime anywhere? When does this general, undercurrent totality and gift interest surface to concrete patterns and experiences? What are the contemporary experiential concretizations of totality interest like? This study purports to qualify the Maussian totality with contemporary experiences.

Upon the insightful Maussian answer, therefore, this book poses another layer of questions that consider the immediate problems in the eyes of the plasma-donating survivors: life in uncertainties and liminality stemming from COVID-19. To this end, the book extends Mauss to the sociology of liminality and its fundamental question – how do people live through liminality? As a result, this book ingeniously formulates the following questions. How do COVID-19 survivors, who, upon infection, have each lost totality as an individual being – they were seen as lacking in some ways – and become marginalized, live through liminality? What does plasma donation have to do with their living through liminality? These questions are empirically more legitimate and immediate to donors' life experiences compared to the Maussian question explicitly targeted at gifts (i.e., why bother to give?) because the questions zoom in on the apparent gift-giving among survivors and yet do not assume their act as gift-giving a priori. While some donors give their plasma self-proclaimingly as gifts, others may well give it simply as a way of continuing their unarticulated daily existence. In this sense, these questions address the most urgent, existential needs of survivors as close as possible to their voices. At the same time, this focus on existential needs does not presumably exclude the possibility that the survivors engage indeed in gift-giving in their efforts to maneuver through liminality.

Narrative Data

This study has conducted interviews from September 2020 to July 2021 with 19 COVID-19 survivors in Korea who have donated blood plasma once or multiple times. They are recruited either by the authors' direct contacts to those whose donation episodes are publicized in the public media and social network services (SNS) or by the invitation of a practicing nurse at the Korea University's Ansan Medical Center to those who have donated at the facility which was one of the only four plasma donation-accepting centers – and the only center in and around the Seoul metropolitan area – in the country during the period. These interviewees have tested positive for the virus during the first months of the pandemic – mainly from February to April 2020, been declared to recover after two to six weeks of professional treatments within medical facilities, been released from these facilities, and subsequently have donated convalescent blood plasma between June and December 2020. Therefore, these interviews record people's voices about the early pandemic experiences when things were the most unclear and unknown about COVID-19. The original data collection has been motivated by an overarching sociological interest in how people react to the uncertainties of COVID-19.

While this interest remains current even after three years of "long" COVID, during which people have variably learned to normalize the impacts of COVID-19, this data from the earliest months seems the most relevant to the sociological inquiry on liminality for the following reasons.

In the early few months, the life challenge for the infected to live through COVID-19 has been far more intense than ever. While not many have been infected, many have died of the infection without established medical interventions; essential medical resources, not only heavily equipped facilities but self-care items like masks and hand sanitizers, have run short; the infected have been blamed for the mysterious infection and treated as unbearable threats to the others yet uninfected; contact tracing on who previously contacted the infected and whom the infected later contacted has been mostly tolerated, rewriting the norms of privacy vis-à-vis public safety; religious as well as social gatherings have been all interpreted as the odds for virus infection; infection cases have been judged in moral terms like necessary/unblamable versus unnecessary/careless infections; an ethical distinction has been made between the arguably less reprehensible, small-scale infections involving only a few in one-to-one interactions and the guilty, large-scale infections involving many people; vaccines have not been available yet; repeated infection has been deemed possible; full recovery from infection has been unwarranted; and emergency economic reliefs for the infected have only begun to form. These traits that elevate the COVID-19 uncertainties to the extreme are unique to the early months of 2020.

Each interview runs for approximately 2 hours online via Zoom interfaces. It is guided by a set of semi-structured questions on how people felt about being infected, treated by medical professionals, and released from the quarantine facilities; how they felt about recovering from the infection; how they dealt with everyday matters, friends, family, and coworkers after recovery; what led and drove them to donate plasma in the first place; what causes and meanings their donation developed into, if ever; what impacts their donation (and infection experiences) had on their life at large. Atlas.ti 8 is used for interpretative content analysis (Schreier, 2012). The Korea University IRB has approved the study.

The Argument Ahead

This study contributes to the sociology of liminality by proposing a holistic theory on the ways of liminality that classics have awaited. Our theory has four elements. First, people not uncommonly run into the breakdown of the whole and totality of life – e.g., COVID-19 infection – which manifests in different experiences of turning and remaining liminal (i.e., *original problematic liminality*). Second, people resort to an instance of practice – e.g., plasma donation – consciously as a strategy to live through liminality or unconsciously as an evolving part of living through it. Third, this practice carries variable initial causes and emergent meanings, which makes itself yet another instance of uncertainty and liminality (i.e., *instant liminality*). The ways in which instant liminality plays out – e.g., how many causes and which meanings it carries – depend on how people have turned liminal in the first place by the virus infection and, simultaneously, how the subsequent attempts, conscious and unconscious, to rely on the instant practice are acted out. Fourth, this variation in instant liminality, in turn, has impacts on how people re-accommodate their lives amid original problematic liminality. In brief, our theory formalizes that people live through liminality by way of other instances of liminality. In this process, original problematic liminality shapes particular ways of ensuing instant liminality. At the same time, instant liminality, partly dependent on original liminality and partly contingent on its own processual factors, reconstitutes original liminality. This dialectical operation – i.e., *liminalization,* we suggest – is how terms of liminality can parsimoniously represent all relevant aspects of human existence.

On the substantive front, our holistic theory particularly highlights the fourth element. It argues that the more multiple causes or the more extended series of meanings a person develops in instant liminality, the more likely the person demonstrates that life in original liminality and uncertainty is yet bearable, livable, certain, and even generative. This argument has several implications for the literature. The classics and existing empirical inquiries have suggested without contextualization that liminality can be destructive and generative at once in its consequences. This study adds that liminality as a fundamental life challenge is responded to with another instance of liminality and that the ways in which this instant liminality is practiced produce different consequences of the original liminality, varying from being destructive to generative. When instant liminality proceeds as a static, simple practice, it tends to make destructive but not generative effects of original liminality. When instant liminality plays out as a dynamic, complex practice, it induces generative consequences as well as destructive ones. Regarding the generative process, this study proposes an ingenious twofold link between original and instant liminalities. First, as far as people experience an instant practice like plasma donation as developing *multiple, unpredicted meanings* and, nonetheless, *being concretely and evidently present*, they tend to normalize the original liminality laden with conflicting, unfathomable uncertainties amid COVID-19 as something that is real, livable, and generative. Second, while people are experiencing multiple meanings and elements joined together in instant liminality, they sometimes learn that *uncertain, personal* meanings are bound up with *collective, supra-individual certainties.* As much as the instant liminality is experienced to convey both personal uncertainties and collective certainty, people learn to accept life amid the original liminality as one that can harbor certainty amid many uncertainties. To illustrate it, when people experience that personal worries about virus infection and plasma donations end up with social gratitude for their convalescent donations, they learn to countenance other worries and disorders during COVID-19 with hopes and orders, if unspecified and unspeakable at times.

This study opens up another sociological discourse. By making Turner's and van Gennep's sociology of liminality engage with the Maussian sociology of gift-giving through the contemporary case amid COVID-19, this study rejuvenates the Maussian notion of individual existence and agency as totality. Mauss stresses as early as in the 1920s that "after having of necessity divided things up too much, and abstracted from them, the sociologists must strive to reconstitute the whole. By so doing they will discover rewarding facts" (Mauss, 1990 [1925], p. 80). Rewarding facts in this quote refer to revelations of individuality and agency as totality. In search of such rewarding facts, Mauss does not call for attention to macro-level instances of sociality, such as structure and system per se, but invites inquiries on how many "needs" and "inclinations" (Mauss, 1990 [1925], p. 76) people try to satisfy and actually meet, for example, in his own treatment of the gift. One can respond to Mauss's call by investigating other empirical categories of totality, such as money, ritual, time, and honor, as Mauss himself insinuates in the book, or by continuing the inquiry on the gift in new lights. This study takes the latter direction, as it has translated Mauss's call into the question about when the seemingly general totality – i.e., the gift – that is therefore elusive to always particular human experiential capacities reveals itself and in what partialities.

Elaborating on what plasma donations mean during the pandemic, this study shows that donations that Mauss calls *totality* are experiences of *liminality*. It suggests that individuals experience the Maussian totality – i.e., the riches and complexity of individual existence – often in terms of liminality. This implies that, conversely, liminal experiences that are often devastating and disorderly attest to people the totality and riches of individual existence. Individual existence becomes as liminal as it is total. Liminality does not occur without totality, although totality does not always produce liminality. Put in another way, the experiential endeavors among plasma donors provide a unique window through which we observe that Mauss's seemingly structuralist and transcendental proposition of totality never divorces the processual and immanent experiences of liminality. It is reassuring to see a similar emphasis on *process* theory and social *drama* when Turner's sociology of liminality purports to master social *structure* (Turner, 1985).

In addition, these propositions about the relationship between totality and liminality serve as an answer to the very plausible question about the relationship between *gifts* and *rites of passage* (Silber, 2018), which is prevalent in contemporary everyday practice – e.g., presents at births, commencements, retirements, deaths, etc. This study agrees with Silber that Mauss has left unaccounted what rites of passage may mean in gift relations and that van Gennep has given little attention to how gifts relate to rites of passage. These are surprising blind spots of both scholars, given that van Gennep's book is full of the descriptions of gifts associated with rites of passage, such as *cadeaux, presents, dons*, and *donations religieuses*, tributes, hospitality, banquets, and feasts; salutations, exchanges, and ceremonial exchanges. As for Mauss, the description of various gift exchanges is often embedded in rituals and ceremonies that are yet undertheorized. While van Gennep elaborates on liminality based on rituals and yet neglects totality inherent to the gift, unheeding the possible link between liminality and totality, Mauss is short on liminality and long on totality. In order to resolve this mismatch, Silber revisits Mauss and proposes that most gift relations in Mauss can be reconceptualized as van Gennep's liminality experiences. Thus, Silber argues in a conceptual manner that van Gennep may well have preceded Mauss's totality theory of gifts in terms of his liminality theory. This study agrees that gifts – i.e., totality – do not only appear in rites of passage – i.e., liminality – but they are themselves rites of passage in nature. For instance, gift-making is a succession of well-defined acts, undefined pauses, and intervals in between. In resonance, this study further argues that crises that the pandemic has created are crises on individual existence as a total being, that gift practices accompany these liminal moments as a way of living through them, that gift practices that are so far known as totality practices mostly have traits of liminality, and finally that people counteract liminality with another instance of liminality with different consequences depending on how the instant liminality unfolds (cf. Szakolczai, 2017).

The following chapters are organized to these ends. Chapter 1 explicates the sociology of liminality by visiting the two most prominent classical theorists, Arnold van Gennep and Victor Turner. It focuses on conceptualizing three essential aspects of liminality experience and how they can be applied to people's lives during COVID-19. It also foreshadows how the COVID-19 experiences can renew the sociology of liminality. The subsequent empirical descriptions in Chapters 2–4 are largely twofold. After exploring themes freely emerging from participant narratives to interview questions, interpretative content analysis reconstitutes the ways of liminality into three main themes such as "turning liminal" (Chapter 2), "plasma donations" (Chapter 3), and "life reassembled" (Chapter 4), each of which is composed of several sub-themes. Each chapter represents those themes analytically in the form of qualitative coding frames, that is, relations of main themes and sub-themes. Simultaneously, these chapters altogether synthesize how experiences of turning liminal, people's responses to them, and plasma donations affect the ways in which life amid liminality is being reassembled. Conclusion summarizes the preceding empirical chapters by formalizing the argument that original problematic liminality – i.e., liminality as a problematic like the COVID-19 liminality – is lived through effectively by an instance of liminality – i.e., liminality as a solution like blood plasma donations. It discusses the implications of this argument for the sociologies of liminality and gifts and the promises of liminality and the gift as the due sociological languages available to people's lived experiences in different contexts.

References

Aguilar, F. V. Jr (2018 [1999]). Ritual passage and the reconstruction of selfhood in international labour migration. *SOJOURN: Journal of Social Issues in Southeast Asia, 33*, S87–S130, https://doi.org/10.1355/sj33-Se

Appiah, K. A. (2020). Is it ok to ask patients for their plasma? *The New York Times.* https://www.nytimes.com/2020/08/18/magazine/is-it-ok-to-ask-patients-for-their-plasma.html?searchResultPosition=2

Atanasova, L. (2019). The Korean Demilitarized Zone (DMZ) as liminal space and heterotopia. *Sociological Problems, 51*, 410–424.

Berger, P. L., & Luckmann, T. (1991 [1967]). *The social construction of reality: A treatise in the sociology of knowledge.* Penguin Books.

Bloch, E. M., Shoham, S., Casadevall, A., Sachais, B. S., Shaz, B., Winters, J. L., Van Buskirk, C., Grossman, B. J., Joyner, M., & Henderson, J. P. (2020). Deployment of convalescent plasma for the prevention and treatment of COVID-19. *The Journal of Clinical Investigation, 130*(6), 2757–2765.

Bourdieu, P. (2000). *Pascalian meditations* (R. Nice, Trans.). Stanford University Press.

Brown, P. (1995). Naming and framing: The social construction of diagnosis and illness, *Journal of Health and Social Behavior, 35*, 34–52, http://www.jstor.org/stable/2626956

Coleman, J. S. (1990). *Foundations of social theory.* Harvard University Press. https://books.google.co.kr/books?id=a4Dl8tiX4b8C

Conrad, P. (2005). The shifting engines of medicalization, *Journal of Health and Social Behavior, 46*, 3–14, http://search.proquest.com/docview/60527 599?accountid=14657http://sfx.lib.uchicago.edu/sfx_local?url_ver=Z39.88-2004&rft_val_fmt=info:ofi/fmt:kev:mtx:journal&genre=article&sid=ProQ: ProQ%3Asocabsshell&atitle=The+Shifting+Engines+of+Medicalization&title= Journal+of+Health+and+Social+Behavior&issn=00221465&date=2005-03-01&vo lume=46&issue=1&spage=3&au=Conrad%2C+Peter&isbn=&jtitle=Journal+ of+Health+and+Social+Behavior&btitle=&rft_id=info:eric/

Cormier, N. R., Gallo-Cruz, S. R., & Beard, R. L. (2017). Navigating the new, transplanted self: How recipients manage the cognitive risks of organ transplantation. *Sociology of Health & Illness, 39*(8), 1496–1513. https://doi.org/10.1111/1467-9566.12610

Crowder, L. A., Steele, W. R., Goodhue, E., Lasky, B., & Young, P. P. (2023). COVID-19 convalescent plasma donors: Unique motivations in unique times. *Transfusion, 63*(4), 703–710.

Czarniawska, B., & Mazza, C. (2003). Consulting as a liminal space. *Human Relations, 56*(3), 267–290. https://doi.org/10.1177/0018726703056003612

Ekins, R., & King, D. (1999). Towards a sociology of transgendered bodies. *The Sociological Review, 47*(3), 580–602. https://doi.org/10.1111/1467-954X.00185

Forss, A., Tishelman, C., Widmark, C., & Sachs, L. (2004). Women's experiences of cervical cellular changes: An unintentional transition from health to liminality? *Sociology of Health & Illness, 26*(3), 306–325. https://doi.org/10.1111/j.1467-9566.2004.00392.x

Garces, C., & Jones, A. (2009). Mauss Redux: From Warfare's human toll to "L'homme total." *Anthropological Quarterly, 82*(1), 279–309. http://www.jstor.org/stable/25488266

Ghorashi, H., de Boer, M., & ten Holder, F. (2017). Unexpected agency on the threshold: Asylum seekers narrating from an asylum seeker centre. *Current Sociology, 66*(3), 373–391. https://doi.org/10.1177/0011392117703766

Gofman, A. (1998). A vague but suggestive concept: The 'Total social Fact'. In W. James & N. J. Allen (Eds.), *Marcel Mauss: A centenary tribute* (pp. 63–70). Berghahn Books.

Harmon, A. (2020). 'You could lick the benches': Life for the first wave of U.S. survivors. *The New York Times.* https://www.nytimes.com/2020/04/11/us/coronavirus-survivors.html?searchResultPosition=1

Horvath, A., Thomassen, B., & Wydra, H. (2015). *Breaking boundaries: Varieties of liminality.* Berghahn Books.

Huaxia. (2021). China establishes COVID-19 convalescent-plasma supply network. *Xinhua.* http://www.xinhuanet.com/english/2021-06/10/c_1310000986.htm

Jerolmack, C. (2013). Who's worried about turkeys? How 'organisational silos' impede zoonotic disease surveillance. *Sociology of Health & Illness, 35*(2), 200–212. https://doi.org/10.1111/j.1467-9566.2012.01501.x

Jones, K. E., Patel, N. G., Levy, M. A., Storeygard, A., Balk, D., Gittleman, J. L., & Daszak, P. (2008). Global trends in emerging infectious diseases. *Nature, 451*(7181), 990–993. https://doi.org/10.1038/nature06536

Jordan, J., Price, J., & Prior, L. (2015). Disorder and disconnection: Parent experiences of liminality when caring for their dying child. *Sociology of Health & Illness, 37*(6), 839–855. https://doi.org/10.1111/1467-9566.12235

Joseph, J., Liamputtong, P., & Brodribb, W. (2019). From liminality to vitality: Infant feeding beliefs among refugee mothers from Vietnam and Myanmar. *Qualitative Health Research, 30*(8), 1171–1182. https://doi.org/10.1177/1049732318825147

Kim, K. (2021). March 'beyond' the life: Ritual walk for the death in the 'Liminality' of Covid-19 [생명 '너머의' 행진: 코로나19 '리미널리티' 속 죽음에 대한 걷기의례]. *Cross-Cultural Studies, 27*(2), 5–68.

Kim, G. H., Lee, S.-Y., & Park, S. J. (2020). Between the 'Employed' and the 'Unemployed': A case study of Korean youth turnover ['취업'과 '실업'의 사이에서: 청년이직에 대한 질적연구]. *Korea Social Policy Review, 27*(4), 49–85.

Kosar, A., & Kasapoglu, A. (2021). Sociology of everyday life with uncertainty and differences during the COVID-19 pandemic process: The case of Turkey retirees association. *Advances in Applied Sociology, 11*(12), 747–772.

Kupferschmidt, K. (2020). Scientists put survivors' blood plasma to the test. *Science, 368*(6494), 922–923. https://doi.org/doi:10.1126/science.368.6494.922

Lamond, I. R., & Moss, J. (Eds.). (2020). *Liminality and critical event studies: Borders, boundaries, and contestation.* Springer Nature.

Lamont, M., & Molnár, V. (2002). The study of boundaries in the social sciences. *Annual Review of Sociology, 28*, 167–195, https://doi.org/10.1146/annurev. soc.28.110601.141107

Lasky, B., Goodhue Meyer, E., Steele, W. R., Crowder, L. A., & Young, P. P. (2021). COVID-19 convalescent plasma donor characteristics, product disposition, and comparison with standard apheresis donors. *Transfusion, 61*(5), 1471–1478. https://doi.org/10.1111/trf.16286

Li, L., Yang, R., Wang, J., Lv, Q., Ren, M., Zhao, L., Chen, H., Xu, H., Xie, S., Xie, J., Lin, H., Li, W., Fang, P., Gong, L., Wang, L., Wu, Y., & Liu, Z. (2020). Feasibility of a pilot program for COVID-19 convalescent plasma collection in Wuhan, China. *Transfusion, 60*(8), 1773–1777. https://doi.org/10.1111/trf. 15921

Lupton, D. (1995). *The imperative of health: Public health the regulated body.* Sage.

MacArtney, J. I., Broom, A., Kirby, E., Good, P., & Wootton, J. (2017). The liminal and the parallax: Living and dying at the end of life. *Qualitative Health Research, 27*(5), 623–633. https://doi.org/10.1177/1049732315618938

Mackintosh, N., & Armstrong, N. (2020). Understanding and managing uncertainty in health care: Revisiting and advancing sociological contributions. *Sociology of Health & Illness, 42*(S1), 1–20. https://doi.org/10.1111/1467-9566.13160

Maheshwari, A., Varshney, M., Bajpai, M., Raizada, N., & Sharma, T. (2022). An exploratory study of the differences in attitudes and motives regarding COVID-19 plasma donation. *Acta Medica Lituanica, 29*(1), 69.

Malksoo, M. (2015). The challenge of liminality for international relations theory. In A. Horvath, B. Thomassen, & H. Wydra (Eds.), *Breaking boundaries: Varieties of liminality* (pp. 226–243). Berghahn.

Masser, B. M., Ferguson, E., Thorpe, R., Lawrence, C., Davison, T. E., Hoad, V., & Gosbell, I. B. (2021). Motivators of and barriers to becoming a COVID-19 convalescent plasma donor: A survey study. *Transfusion Medicine, 31*(3), 176–185.

Mauss, M. (1973 [1934]). Techniques of the body. *Economy and Society, 2*, 70–88, https://doi.org/10.1080/03085147300000003

Mauss, M. (1985 [1938]). A category of the human mind: The notion of person, the notion of self. In M. Carrithers, S. Collins, & S. Lukes (Eds.), *The category of the person: Anthropology, philosophy, history* (pp. 1–25). Cambridge University Press.

Mauss, M. (1990 [1925]). *The gift: The form and reason for exchange in archaic societies* (W. D. Halls, Trans.). W. W. Norton.

Menjívar, C. (2006). Liminal legality: Salvadoran and Guatemalan immigrants' lives in the United States. *American Journal of Sociology, 111*(4), 999–1037. https://doi.org/10.1086/499509

Mountz, A. (2011). Where asylum-seekers wait: Feminist counter-topographies of sites between states. *Gender, Place & Culture, 18*(3), 381–399. https://doi.org/ 10.1080/0966369X.2011.566370

Mu, X. (2020). China focus: Cured coronavirus patients donate plasma to save more. *Xinhua.* http://www.xinhuanet.com/english/2020-02/16/c_138789290.htm

Murphy, M., Estcourt, L., Grant-Casey, J., & Dzik, S. (2020). International survey of trials of convalescent plasma to treat COVID-19 infection. *Transfusion Medicine Reviews*, *34*(3), 151–157.

O'Reilly, Z. (2018). 'Living Liminality': Everyday experiences of asylum seekers in the 'Direct Provision' system in Ireland. *Gender, Place & Culture*, *25*(6), 821–842. https://doi.org/10.1080/0966369X.2018.1473345

Pant, S., Bagha, R., & McGill, S. (2021). International plasma collection practices: Project report. *Canadian Journal of Health Technologies*, *1*(12), 1–38.

Pozzo, M., & Ghorashi, H. (2021). How liminality enhances conviviality through multilingual co-creations: Young refugees in the Netherlands. *Current Sociology*, *70*(5), 682–702. https://doi.org/10.1177/0011392120932933

Rebughini, P. (2021). A sociology of anxiety: Western modern legacy and the COVID-19 outbreak. *International Sociology*, *36*(4), 554–568. https://doi.org/10.1177/0268580921993325

Roberts, D. J., Miflin, G., & Estcourt, L. (2020). Convalescent plasma for COVID-19: Back to the future. *Transfusion Medicine (Oxford, England)*, *30*(3), 174.

Rubin, R. (2020). Testing an old therapy against a new disease: Convalescent plasma for COVID-19. *Journal of the American Medical Association*, *323*(21), 2114–2117. https://doi.org/10.1001/jama.2020.7456

Rubin, R. (2022). Once viewed as a promising COVID-19 treatment, convalescent plasma falls out of favor. *Journal of the American Medical Association*, *327*(12), 1115–1116. https://doi.org/10.1001/jama.2022.3214

Schreier, M. (2012). *Qualitative content analysis in practice*. Sage Publications.

Scott, S., Prior, L., Wood, F., & Gray, J. (2005). Repositioning the patient: The implications of being 'at risk'. *Social Science & Medicine*, *60*(8), 1869–1879. https://doi.org/10.1016/j.socscimed.2004.08.020

Shim, J.-M. (2022). Patient agency: Manifestations of individual agency among people with health problems. *SAGE Open*, *12*(1). https://doi.org/10.1177/21582440221085010

Silber, I. F. (2009). Bourdieu's gift to gift theory: An unacknowledged trajectory. *Sociological Theory*, *27*(2), 173–190. http://www.jstor.org/stable/40376130

Silber, I. F. (2018). Gifts in rites of passage or gifts as rites of passage? Standing at the threshold between van Gennep and Marcel Mauss. *Journal of Classical Sociology*, *18*(4), 348–360. https://doi.org/10.1177/1468795X18789017

Silver, I. (1996). Role transitions, objects, and identity. *Symbolic Interaction*, *19*(1), 1–20. https://doi.org/10.1525/si.1996.19.1.1

Star, S. L., & Griesemer, J. R. (1989). Institutional ecology, 'Translations' and boundary objects: Amateurs and professionals in Berkeley's Museum of vertebrate zoology, 1907–39. *Social Studies of Science*, *19*(3), 387–420. https://doi.org/10.1177/030631289019003001

Suárez-Orozco, C., Yoshikawa, H., Teranishi, R. T., & Suárez-Orozco, M. M. (2011). Growing up in the shadows: The developmental implications of unauthorized status. *Harvard Educational Review*, *81*(3), 438–472, 619–620.

Szakolczai, A. (2017). Permanent (trickster) liminality: The reasons of the heart and of the mind. *Theory & Psychology*, *27*(2), 231–248. https://doi.org/10.1177/0959354317694095

Terada, M., Kutsuna, S., Togano, T., Saito, S., Kinoshita, N., Shimanishi, Y., Suzuki, T., Miyazato, Y., Inada, M., & Nakamoto, T. (2021). How we secured a COVID-19 convalescent plasma procurement scheme in Japan. *Transfusion*, *61*(7), 1998–2007.

Thomas, K., & Weiland, N. (2021). The COVID-19 plasma boom is over: What did we learn from it? *New York Times*.

Timmermans, S., & Buchbinder, M. (2010). Patients-in-waiting: Living between sickness and health in the genomics era. *Journal of Health and Social Behavior*, *51*(4), 408–423. https://doi.org/10.1177/0022146510386794

Timmermans, S., & Haas, S. (2008). Towards a sociology of disease, *Sociology of Health and Illness*, *30*, 659–676, https://doi.org/10.1111/j.1467-9566.2008.01097.x

Turner, E. (1985). Prologue: From the Ndembu to Broadway. In E. Turner (Ed.), *On the edge of the Bush: Anthropology as experience* (pp. 1–15). University of Arizona Press.

Turner, V. (1967). Betwixt and between: The liminal period in rites de passage. In V. Turner (Ed.), *The forest of symbols: Aspects of Ndembu ritual* (pp. 93–111). Cornell University Press.

Turner, V. (1982). *From ritual to theatre: The human seriousness of play*. PAJ Publications.

Turner, V. (1985a). The anthropology of performance. In E. Turner (Ed.), *On the edge of the Bush: Anthropology as experience* (pp. 177–204). University of Arizona Press.

Turner, V. (1985b). Epilogue: Are there universals of performance in myth, ritual, and drama? In E. Turner (Ed.), *On the edge of the bush: Anthropology as experience* (pp. 291–301). University of Arizona Press.

Turner, V. (1967). *The forest of symbols: Aspects of Ndembu ritual* (Vol. 101). Cornell University Press.

Turner, V. (1991 [1969]). *The ritual process: Structure and anti-structure*. Cornell University Press.

Turner, V., & Turner, E. (1978). *Image and pilgrimage in Christian culture: Anthropological perspective*. Columbia University Press.

van Gennep, A. (1960 [1909]). *The rites of passage* (M. B. Vizedom & G. L. Caffee, Trans.). University of Chicago Press.

Wade, J., Dent, E. A., Wooten, M. S., Moosavi, M., Butler, H., Lough, C., Verkerke, H., Kamili, N. A., Maier, C. L., Josephson, C. D., Roback, J. D., Stowell, S. R., & Sullivan, H. C. (2021). COVID-19 convalescent plasma donor recruitment experience from the perspective of a hospital transfusion medicine service. *Transfusion*, *61*(7), 2213–2215. https://doi.org/10.1111/trf.16448

Ward, P. R. (2020). A sociology of the COVID-19 pandemic: A commentary and research agenda for sociologists. *Journal of Sociology*, *56*(4), 726–735. https://doi.org/10.1177/1440783320939682

Ward, P. R., Foley, K., Meyer, S. B., Thomas, J., Huppatz, E., Olver, I., Miller, E. R., & Lunnay, B. (2022). Uncertainty, fear and control during COVID-19 … or … making a safe boat to survive rough seas: The lived experience of women in South Australia during early COVID-19 lockdowns. In P. R. Brown & J. O. Zinn (Eds.), *COVID-19 and the sociology of risk and uncertainty: Studies of social phenomena and social theory across 6 continents* (pp. 167–190). Springer International Publishing. https://doi.org/10.1007/978-3-030-95167-2_7

Wendel, S., Land, K., Devine, D. V., Daly, J., Bazin, R., Tiberghien, P., Lee, C. K., Arora, S., Patidar, G. K., & Khillan, K. (2021). Lessons learned in the collection of convalescent plasma during the COVID-19 pandemic. *Vox Sanguinis, 116*(8), 872–879.

Wilson, M. (2002). 'I am the prince of pain, for I am a princess in the Brain': Liminal transgender identities, narratives and the elimination of ambiguities. *Sexualities, 5*(4), 425–448. https://doi.org/10.1177/1363460702005004003

Wiltshire, G., Clarke, N. J., Phoenix, C., & Bescoby, C. (2020). Organ transplant Recipients' experiences of physical activity: Health, self-care, and transliminality. *Qualitative Health Research, 31*(2), 385–398. https://doi.org/10.1177/1049732320967915

Wimark, T. (2021). Homemaking and perpetual liminality among queer refugees. *Social & Cultural Geography, 22*(5), 647–665. https://doi.org/10.1080/14649365.2019.1619818

Yan. (2020). China focus: China urges plasma donation among cured coronavirus patients. *Xinhua.* http://www.news.cn/english/2020-02/15/c_138787205.htm

Zinn, J. O. (2021). Introduction: Towards a sociology of pandemics. *Current Sociology, 69*(4), 435–452. https://doi.org/10.1177/00113921211020771

1 Ways of Liminality

The sociological literature describes various ways in which individuals encounter liminality in the first place, how they live with it once encountered, and what consequences they go through. Drawing on the literature from classics to contemporary studies in the discipline, this chapter constitutes several expectations that will ultimately be expanded into a new theory of liminality when the Korean case is elaborated in the subsequent empirical analysis.

van Gennep's Initiation: From Rituals to Liminality

The sociological and anthropological origin of the inquiry on liminality is documented in van Gennep's (1960 [1909]) classic book *The Rites of Passage* (Silber, 2018; Szakolczai, 2009; Thomassen, 2009, 2012). There seems to be a temporal distance between this classic and the current experiences of coronavirus disease-2019 (COVID-19). Nevertheless, this study finds a resonance between the two and expects that the current experiences will not only be elucidated by the theory; they will also renew and advance the existing theory in a new direction. Amid COVID-19, individuals find themselves in situations challenging established ways and forms of life and existence. Accordingly, people forcibly or voluntarily invest in new and experimental ways and, furthermore, the processually unfolding moments of life themselves. van Gennep's interest in rituals originates in the same commitment to the processual experiences of life, or "living" social facts, as opposed to "dead" facts (Thomassen, 2009).

van Gennep posits that rituals are instances of living facts or facts that are flowing and living. Therefore, van Gennep collects ethnographical studies of ceremonies, rites, and magico-religious acts in the book. He calls these rites the rites of passage and transition. He classifies them into subgroups, such as rites for the passage/transition of individual and collective actors from one status/stage to another (e.g., birth and death) and rites for the transition of time (e.g., harvest and new year) and the

DOI: 10.4324/9781003493723-2

transition of space from one to another. Along with the classification, the book proposes a theorization about the general structure of these rituals. Before one jumps to his ultimate formalization of this universal structure, it is critical to locate van Gennep's answer to two fundamental questions in order to properly contextualize the book's sociological bearings on the current inquiry. So, we pose the following questions: How is it that van Gennep fashions his interest in rituals as that in living facts (but not others)? Once into rituals, why is he preoccupied with passage and transition?

The book collects and reinterprets the accumulated ethnographical studies of rites because rites are deemed important for the "existence" and "life" of individuals and collectivities (ibid., pp. 2–3). The ways in which rites help existence and life are found to be intriguingly twofold. First, rites confirm and protect existence by putting life processes within established categories, times, and spaces that are not only natural-physical but also social-cultural. Rites enable individuals to pass from "one defined position to another which is equally well defined" (ibid., p. 3). In addition, rites help existence and life by providing ways to place life processes outside these established entities and categories but within the flow of a ritual. An elaboration should help understand this seemingly contradictory presentation on the relationship between categories and existence.

In addressing what enables life and existence, the book considers "differences," different "categories," "separate social groupings," and "groups and subgroups" to be fundamental to human existence and life (ibid., p. 1). In particular, the life of an individual or a collectivity is formulated as "a series of passages" from one category to another (ibid., p. 2). Life is defined as a succession of different entities, which is a temporal rendition of plurality and multiplicity. The book also states, "life itself means to separate and to be reunited, to change form and condition, to die and to be reborn. It is to act and to cease, to wait and rest, and then to begin acting again, but in a different way" (ibid., p. 189); life is to "cross thresholds" and to synchronically "join individuals in other sections" (ibid., p. 189). "This (already) complex world of the living" is further joined by "the world preceding life" and "the one which follows death" (ibid., p. 189). "Transitions … are looked on as implicit in the very fact of existence, so that a man's life … is a succession of stages" (ibid., p. 3). These stages can be temporal and spatial. In sum, life and existence are defined to be within categories and between categories; they consist of categories, anti-categories, and non-categories.

This formulation of life in terms of multiple, fundamental categories is no more problematic than the fact that there are tensions and conflicts between one category and another – e.g., between a child and an adult. In order to navigate through these necessarily multiple and yet potentially incompatible categories, one needs intermediate categories or non-categories that make the transition across categories smooth and possible.

Magico-religious acts, or rituals, produce and exist as intermediate categories, non-categories, and unknowns – that help incompatible knowns exist side by side. To this extent, rituals are aptly called the rites that are for and of passage and transition.

At the same time, however, rituals are far from being unproblematic. A ritual is functional and effective for passage and transition just because it is fraught with tensions between categories and intermediate, in-between categories – e.g., between childhood and adulthood on the one hand and adolescence/puberty on the other – that together constitute the ritual. In addition, a ritual is laden with tensions between categories and non-categories that are all part of the ritual – e.g., between childhood and adulthood on the one hand and, on the other, a whole personhood/being of which the former is only one specific representation; between a social system of roles and its unspecified surrounding non-system (Douglas, 1966). Rituals that involve non-categories do not only make transitions across categories possible; they also readily negate all extant categories and dissolve their status as absolutes and naturals by embodying the possible presence and significance of non-categories and unknowns in juxtaposition. In sum, rituals are a challenge as well as a solution to human existence among multiple categories. They are a threat as well as a help.

van Gennep conceptualizes this dual nature of rituals as liminality. To comprehend this intriguingly contradictory presentation takes an explication of how liminality holds the central place in van Gennep's three-stage, periodic conceptualization of rites. Rites reveal "periodicity" (ibid., p. 3), which is believed to govern human life – i.e., rites of birth, puberty, marriage, death, etc. – and ultimately the universe, as in the rites of the full moon to mark a shift from month to month, the festivals of solstices and equinoxes to mark shifts from season to season, and New Year's festivity to mark a yearly transition. Rites reflect these great "rhythms" in the universe (ibid., p. 194). Interestingly, van Gennep finds, this periodicity in rites can be simplified into "a universal pattern" (i.e., a tripartite structure), although details vary in content. Each rite of passage is composed of "rites of separation, transition rites (or rites of transition), and rites of incorporation" (ibid., p. 11). They are each called preliminal, liminal, and postliminal rites. These rites concern not only an individual life process but also the collective process in the universe. Therefore, all living facts throughout the universe are simplified as various revelations of liminality: Preliminal, liminal, or postliminal existence. As Turner later formalizes, liminality is the essence of living social facts that are sometimes challenging and other times generative.

To the same effect, van Gennep conceptualizes that the extent to which rites of passage – i.e., a synonym for all life and existence – are composed of these three sub-rites varies from one to another. Some rites of life and existence are dominated by sub-rites of transition/liminality, while others are dominated by those of separation (e.g., death) or incorporation (e.g., marriage). Furthermore, a sub-rite of transition/liminality can be "reduplicately" (ibid., p. 11) composed of another series of a separation rite, a transition/liminality rite, and an incorporation rite. This formulation is crucial in the theory. In this formulation, the original sub-rite of liminality, which forms only part of one whole higher-order rite of passage, is simultaneously another whole rite by itself that is, in turn, composed of other lower-order rites of separation, liminality, and incorporation. This formula implies that liminality is not only a part of the whole existence and life, but it is the whole existence and life itself. From this perspective, all life and existence are preliminal, liminal, or postliminal; they are varyingly liminal; they are liminal in different shapes.

After all, what individuals do in everyday life is to deal with and live with liminality. Different actors deal with liminality in different ways. First, people experience life as being composed of separation, betweenness/transition, and incorporation. People sometimes experience separation – the experience of being excluded from established clear-cut categories. Other times, they experience between-ness – the sense of falling in between categories and being placed outside established categories. Still, other times, they experience re-incorporation – the sense of belonging back to established categories. Second, once people experience separation from a known status, some may look to be re-included into another known, established status; alternatively, others may try to adapt to be between known statuses. In the former, people may take liminal moments of life as only a part of the allegedly non-liminal whole life. They treat liminality as a transient experience. In the latter, people take liminality as the ever-present whole, of which non-liminality is only one component. To them, liminality is an underlying, permanent experience.

One only needs to complicate these theoretical suggestions in contemporary empirical cases. People's concern about how to live through liminality during the COVID-19 pandemic – i.e., how to live the transition from pre- to post-pandemic years; how to live these unknown years in between the allegedly pre- and post-pandemic years – is a long-lasting sociological puzzle. Regarding the pandemic, van Gennep implies the following:

van Gennep's Expectation 1. Encountering liminality during the COVID-19 pandemic, people may experience separation, betweenness, or incorporation in relation to existing categories and structures.

van Gennep's Expectation 2. In these experiences, some may seek to remain integrated into known statuses and systems, whereas others may try unknown categories and systems and even settle in liminality in some ways that need to be specified.

Turner's Generalization: Liminality in Everyday Life

This theme of different ways of living liminality emerges in Victor Turner in more detail, who is deemed to rediscover van Gennep's work half a century later and generalize liminal experiences from the rites in small-scale societies to the extra-ritual everyday life matters in large-scale, modern societies (Szakolczai, 2009; Thomassen, 2009, p. vi; Turner, 1991 [1969]). First, Turner defines what liminality means in several qualifications. His definitions are more precise than van Gennep's, and they result from Turner's shift of interest from rituals per se to the human subjects in these rituals. Speaking of the subjects of rites de passage, such as embryos, newborn infants, young adults, and the dead, Turner clarifies the inherent duality of human existence. Human subjects in rituals are often socio-culturally invisible and indefinable while they are physically present (e.g., embryos); other times, they are still well-defined socio-culturally while they are no longer present and gone physically (e.g., the dead). Turner calls these seemingly conflicting, unusual, and unstable experiences of human subjects "liminal" (Turner, 1967, p. 95, 1991 [1969], p. 125). These subjects of liminality are "neither living nor dead from one aspect" and "both living and dead from another." They reveal "ambiguity," "paradox," "confusion," and "sacred poverty (or profanity)" (Turner, 1967, p. 97). In the religious context, liminality refers to a mix of pilgrimage devotion and the market fair, and a "total" field composed of festive play and religious solemnity (Turner & Turner, 1978). It feels like a paradox and a scandal to see, live, and experience what ought not to be present socio-structurally and cognitively; it is a puzzle not to experience personally or corporeally what ought to be present socio-structurally and cognitively. It feels paradoxical and monstrous to pray and play simultaneously in pilgrimage. Turner implies that social actors – both individuals and collectivities – become liminal when they suddenly feel monstrous, scandalous, mysterious, and paradoxical in these manners. Liminal moments are those in which usual frames of reference for action – e.g., established language, categories, and structures – fail to describe the flow of ongoing events.

> *Turner's Expectation 1.* Upon the Covid-19 virus infection that has long remained mysterious diagnostically and prognostically, people may become liminal by losing the usual integrity and whole as individuals; they are likely to turn unwholesome, incomplete, paradoxical, and conflictual across different aspects of life.

Second, therefore, it is an existential concern for liminal subjects – e.g., neophytes and pilgrims in Turner and the infected during the COVID-19 pandemic – to maintain and recognize their existence in some ways throughout the paradoxical and monstrous experiences, which Turner pays closer attention to than van Gennep does. One solution is to subdue liminal experiences to the authority of tradition and conventional categories and dimensions in order to absorb powers for ontological effectiveness from these traditions and categories. This is called the conservative way of obedience and passivity. It is to control and artfully manipulate scandalous and monstrous experiences and succumb to going back to conventional categories and structures. This is part of what rites de passage (Turner, 1967), pilgrimages (Turner & Turner, 1978), and performance arts (Turner, 1985) do to participants by re-incorporating people who are voluntarily or forcibly separated from the established routines and statuses back to those statuses or other established categories. In this way, people live through liminality as if it is transient and transitory.

Turner's Expectation 2-1. In the current context, those who are infected by Covid-19 and later released from medical treatments or cautionary separation in quarantine – i.e., the infected and then recovered – may try to aim for a quick transition from one conventional status – i.e., the ill – to another conventional status – i.e., the healthy.

The other solution is the revolutionary way of equality, egalitarianism, and comradeship among all the liminal subjects by themselves and without reliance on tradition and conventional categories that are non-liminal. Equality refers to the logic of existence in which one liminal entity stands and exists next to another in mutual respect, and one subject of liminality normalizes and enables another liminality in this accompaniment without necessarily getting out of liminality. Rituals are the foremost example in which liminal individuals stand next to one another in companionship and gain recognition not only from one another but also from non-liminal others; furthermore, rituals are by themselves real instances of unlikely companionship – for example, the companionship between the symbolic and the material, between the sacred and the profane, between the spiritual and the material, and between humans and nonhumans like ritual symbols/sacra in Turner. Other examples are pilgrimages that materialize the companionship between prayer and play and between poverty/ordeal and riches/blessing (Turner & Turner, 1978). Performance arts are another example that substantiates the companionship between stage drama and social drama and between front-stage and back-stage (Turner, 1985). It is within – and not outside – these rituals, pilgrimage, and performance arts that are so liminal that paradoxical and monstrous subjects gain ontological recognition. It is a way of effecting one liminal existence by putting it next to another liminal existence. In this way, people live through liminality as if it is permanent and, at least, long-lasting. This way is consonant with Turner's own view that liminality can be permanent as well as transient (Turner, 1991 [1969], pp. 107–109) and that liminality is a constant social fact that has been neglected by social theorists who are eager to unduly consolidate "the 'historicity' of prestigious, unrepeated events" into permanency (Turner & Turner, 1978, p. 1).

> *Turner's Expectation 2-2.* People who are infected with coronaviruses may opt to make the status of being infected normal or less unacceptable rather than trying to move out of the status quickly; people who have survived and recovered from the infection may opt to hold the status of survivorship rather than simply reclaiming the usual status of the healthy.

Third, these liminal experiences and how people respond to them have consequences that are ambivalent and rich: Both destructive and generative; both conservative and revolutionary; both antithetical and synthetical; both self-limiting and self-expanding; and both transition-making and potentiality-making. Turner discusses these consequences on several occasions. Initially, liminality, or the experience of betweenness and instability, enables individuals to take a second look and "reflect" on the usual distinctions between different entities and categories that seem to have been indisputable, such as life versus death, humans versus nonhumans, culture versus nature, cognition versus emotion, and sanctity versus profanity. In reflecting, people now not only come to highlight and "distinguish" these differentials clearly (and even more so sometimes), but they also come to "draw little distinction" and see connectivity and consubstantiality between them by the sheer fact that these differentials do exist together in liminal and yet concrete objects like rituals, ritual symbols (i.e., sacra and the mask) (Turner, 1967, pp. 104–105), pilgrimage, and art performance. In these dual meanings, Turner calls liminal experiences "building" blocks of culture (Turner, 1967, p. 110) that contribute, on one hand, to reproducing and preserving the structure in place that needs only to be revitalized via new energy from anti-structure; on the other, liminal experiences contribute to generating "communitas" defined as "the spontaneous, immediate, concrete," and "total/holistic" order as opposed to "structure" that is the norm-governed, institutionalized, and abstract order that is refuted and destroyed in liminal experiences (Turner & Turner, 1978). "Communitas has an existential quality; it involves the whole man in his relation to other whole men. Structure, on the other hand, has cognitive quality; ... it is a set of classifications" (Turner, 1991 [1969], p. 127). To the extent that liminal experiences provide a realm of total and pure potential in communitas, they build, create, and expand personalities and social structures thereof. They are generative, revolutionary, and self-expanding. On the contrary, to the extent that liminal experiences provide the sense of being outside structure, and being unstructured and chaotic, and to the extent that they highlight and reinforce only what structure has been in place, they introduce uneasiness and the motivation to obey the conventional structure and simply reproduce existential certainties within the structure. They are rather conservative than revolutionary, self-limiting rather than self-expanding.

> *Turner's Expectation 3.* Through infection and recovery, Covid-19 survivors may either revolutionarily transfigure or conservatively reclaim old subjectivities and objectivities. Accordingly, they may experience destruction and regeneration in varying combinations.

Problematics Answered and Unanswered

van Gennep's and Turner's inquiry has generated three related questions that are only partly answered in subsequent empirical studies yet. First, the classics suggest that liminal experiences are fundamental to individual and collective life; contradictorily, those experiences are unique and startling, so social actors often find themselves clueless about what to do. When and in what context do people experience liminal happenings (Thomassen, 2009, p. 20)? In what particularities do people experience the fundamental and universal – thus, potentially unrecognizable – experiences of feeling monstrous, scandalous, paradoxical, undefinable, unstructured, and marginal? Do they ever experience liminality in any real sense? In what particularities does the undercurrent of liminality concretize into everyday experiences? When does liminality become real to people?

Classics themselves point to typical empirical contexts, such as transitions across life stages, pilgrimage journeys, and performance arts that have in common a sense of break and crisis (Turner, 1985). Later studies add contemporary socio-political and economic instances, such as international migration (Aguilar, 2018; Menjívar, 2006), transnational asylum-seeking (Ghorashi et al., 2017; O'Reilly, 2018), international relations/wars (Atanasova, 2019; Malksoo, 2015), emergent work/labor practices (Czarniawska & Mazza, 2003; Kim et al., 2020), human development (Joseph et al., 2019; Silver, 1996; Suárez-Orozco et al., 2011), trans-sexuality (Wilson, 2002; Wimark, 2021), illness/health experiences in health-monitoring technologies (Forss et al., 2004; Scott et al., 2005), organ transplants (Cormier et al., 2017; Wiltshire et al., 2020), end-of-life care (Jordan et al., 2015; MacArtney et al., 2017), and bereavement (Kim, 2021). This list is hardly exhaustive to the extent that every concrete context in which differentials, incongruency, and non-familiarity exist can be an empirical site for particularities of the universal liminality, including the current crisis of COVID-19. This book aims to complicate the fundamental experience of liminality with its particularities during the pandemic by examining how the infected turn liminal and stay liminal and how the recovered remain liminal, not only medical-scientifically but also social-relationally.

Second, the classics suggest that it is an existential challenge for people who have turned or remained liminal to live through liminality and that there can be different ways. While most of those studies that address the first set of questions stop at simply demonstrating that liminality becomes real, some studies further pose this second question. After explicitly identifying liminality as a critical problem for transgender people who manage to hold tight to their unconventional sexuality in the transgender-unfriendly social environment, a study (Wilson, 2002) finds that these people cultivate the way of migrating (i.e., a permanent shift from one to the other binary gender identity) rather than the other three ways, such as oscillating (i.e., repeated temporary shifts between binaries), erasing (i.e., forgetting and denouncing gendered individuality), and transcending (i.e., holding onto gender identity but going beyond the binary limits to an alternative) (Ekins & King, 1999). Another study qualifies the existential challenge amid liminality as how organ recipients redefine their selfhood amid post-transplant physiological risks and social-relational changes in their new body (Cormier et al., 2017). It finds several ways, such as the internal resolve to remain positive and, alternatively, the reliance on familial relations, the divine will, or professional medical expertise. A management study (Czarniawska & Mazza, 2003) that problematizes how part-time management consultants, or the academic-cum-consultants, avoid being trapped in the possible schizophrenic self-understanding finds two rough ways: Some praise the work as the true way of doing management science, while others choose to turn away from the mix to either academe or consulting.

Although informative, these studies do not compare the ways of living liminality that they find with the ways that the classics have already insinuated. Due to this neglect, a promising conceptual dialogue with the classics (Szakolczai, 2017) that liminality can be lived with the help of another instance of liminality – e.g., the heart – or with the instances of conventional, firm categories – e.g., the mind – has been lost in the literature. Theoretical negligence is costly on another front. The studies do not attempt to investigate what consequences each of these ways may produce at the individual and collective levels – i.e., how their lives are reconstituted – which are, according to the classics, the most crucial concerns for liminal subjects and to which the classics do not have rich answers yet. Under scrutiny, studies that do not explicitly address this second question agree with our emphasis on the need for further inquiry. They emphatically show that people in liminality indeed struggle to live through it (Ghorashi et al., 2017; Joseph et al., 2019;

MacArtney et al., 2017) and inadvertently allude to diverse and yet un-organized/undertheorized ways in which people manage to live through liminality – e.g., a mourning walk in response to a bereavement (Kim, 2021), familial and religious relations and arts in dealing with legal liminality (Menjívar, 2006), and physical activities as a way to live the post-transplant bodies (Wiltshire et al., 2020).

Third, the classics suggest that different ways of living liminality may lead to different consequences without a definite theorization. Some subsequent studies explicitly or implicitly examine the consequences of liminal experiences for individualities and collectivities. However, these studies do not situate these consequences in the context of varying ways of living liminality. As a result, they fall short of advancing the classical suggestion. A study on the developmental consequences of liminality among undocumented immigrants demonstrates multiple negative outcomes without portraying how liminality is responded to in different possible ways (Suárez-Orozco et al., 2011). Thus, while producing the impression that liminality generates only negative consequences, this study fails to give any triangulation point at which one can compare this result with an antithetical finding that illegal immigrants are not without producing positive life experiences amid liminality, which lacks a contextual qualification as well (Pozzo & Ghorashi, 2021). The finding (Wiltshire et al., 2020) that physical activities help organ transplant recipients, who remain liminal between life and death and between self and other, to attain physical and psychological well-being does not tell much about what physical activities feature as one of the possible ways to live through liminality.

While some studies report mixed findings on the consequences, they regrettably do not provide a long-awaited theorization on where these divergent consequences come from. A study on illegal immigrants (Menjívar, 2006) finds that the immigrants undergo amid liminal legality not only devastating life consequences but also resilient agency, while the study does not examine the classics-suggested relationship between the way of living liminality and its consequences. A study on breastfeeding (Joseph et al., 2019) finds that the liminal entity of breastmilk produces vitality as well as vulnerability to mothers and infants without a contextualization of the ways in which breastfeeding is lived. A study on globalization (Szakolczai, 2016) implies that the consequences that liminality brings about can be positive – i.e., social flourishing defined as the simultaneous experience of both the sacred and the profane – and negative – i.e., the dark-age globalization and expansion – without due contextualization.

This book provides an innovative model on the ways of liminality that cut through all these three heretofore disconnected aspects of liminality. Three chapters to come elaborate on how these theoretical possibilities are qualified in real experiences. First, themes of liminality materialize in different shapes in which people represent their experiences of falling ill to the coronaviruses and their response inside and outside the professional medical treatments (Chapter 2). Second, upon being declared by the health authority to have recovered, people decide to donate plasma in two fashions. Some present it consciously as an effective way to deal with the problematic liminality that the virus infection has produced. In contrast, others donate it without such expectations and, instead, out of situational exigencies amid COVID-19. Either way, people ascribe various meanings and causes to plasma donation. Some develop a dynamically evolving set of emergent meanings from donation in addition to a set of initial causes. Others reveal only a static, fixed set of initial meanings that underlie donations. When donors go through evolving meanings, this semantic evolution varies across donors in quantity – i.e., how many meanings – and in quality – i.e., which meanings and in what evolving sequences. When donors reveal static meanings, variations are discovered in quantity. These diverse aspects are described in personal voices in Chapter 3. Third, depending on what semantic processes donors go through in plasma donation, life amid COVID-19 is represented differently. The more multiple causes or the more extended series of meanings a person develops in plasma donation, the more likely the person demonstrates that life amid the COVID-19-produced uncertainty is yet bearable, livable, certain, and even generative (Chapter 4).

References

Aguilar, F. V. Jr (2018 [1999]). Ritual passage and the reconstruction of selfhood in international labour migration. *SOJOURN: Journal of Social Issues in Southeast Asia, 33*, S87–S130. https://doi.org/10.1355/sj33-Se

Atanasova, L. (2019). The Korean demilitarized zone (DMZ) as liminal space and heterotopia. *Sociological Problems, 51*, 410–424.

Cormier, N. R., Gallo-Cruz, S. R., & Beard, R. L. (2017). Navigating the new, transplanted self: How recipients manage the cognitive risks of organ transplantation. *Sociology of Health & Illness, 39*(8), 1496–1513. https://doi.org/10.1111/1467-9566.12610

Czarniawska, B., & Mazza, C. (2003). Consulting as a liminal space. *Human Relations, 56*(3), 267–290. https://doi.org/10.1177/0018726703056003612

Douglas, M. (1966). *Purity and danger: An analysis of concept of pollution and taboo*. Routledge.

Ekins, R., & King, D. (1999). Towards a sociology of transgendered bodies. *The Sociological Review, 47*(3), 580–602. https://doi.org/10.1111/1467-954X.00185

Forss, A., Tishelman, C., Widmark, C., & Sachs, L. (2004). Women's experiences of cervical cellular changes: An unintentional transition from health to liminality. *Sociology of Health & Illness, 26*(3), 306–325. https://doi.org/10.1111/j.1467-9566.2004.00392.x

Ghorashi, H., de Boer, M., & ten Holder, F. (2017). Unexpected agency on the threshold: Asylum seekers narrating from an asylum seeker centre. *Current Sociology*, *66*(3), 373–391. https://doi.org/10.1177/0011392117703766

Jordan, J., Price, J., & Prior, L. (2015). Disorder and disconnection: Parent experiences of liminality when caring for their dying child. *Sociology of Health & Illness*, *37*(6), 839–855. https://doi.org/10.1111/1467-9566.12235

Joseph, J., Liamputtong, P., & Brodribb, W. (2019). From liminality to vitality: Infant feeding beliefs among refugee mothers from Vietnam and Myanmar. *Qualitative Health Research*, *30*(8), 1171–1182. https://doi.org/10.1177/1049732318825147

Kim, G. H., Lee, S.-Y., & Park, S. J. (2020). Between the 'Employed' and the 'Unemployed': A case study of Korean youth turnover ['취업'과 '실업'의 사이에서: 청년이직에 대한 질적연구]. *Korea Social Policy Review*, *27*(4), 49–85.

Kim, K. (2021). March 'beyond' the life: Ritual walk for the death in the 'Liminality' of COVID-19 [생명 '너머의' 행진: 코로나19 '리미널리티' 속 죽음에 대한 걷기의례]. *Cross-Cultural Studies*, *27*(2), 5–68.

MacArtney, J. I., Broom, A., Kirby, E., Good, P., & Wootton, J. (2017). The liminal and the parallax: Living and dying at the end of life. *Qualitative Health Research*, *27*(5), 623–633. https://doi.org/10.1177/1049732315618938

Malksoo, M. (2015). The challenge of liminality for international relations theory. In A. Horvath, B. Thomassen, & H. Wydra (Eds.), *Breaking boundaries: Varieties of liminality* (pp. 226–243). Berghahn.

Menjívar, C. (2006). Liminal legality: Salvadoran and Guatemalan immigrants' lives in the United States. *American Journal of Sociology*, *111*(4), 999–1037. https://doi.org/10.1086/499509

O'Reilly, Z. (2018). 'Living Liminality': Everyday experiences of asylum seekers in the 'Direct Provision' system in Ireland. *Gender, Place & Culture*, *25*(6), 821–842. https://doi.org/10.1080/0966369X.2018.1473345

Pozzo, M., & Ghorashi, H. (2021). How liminality enhances conviviality through multilingual co-creations: Young refugees in the Netherlands. *Current Sociology*, https://doi.org/10.1177/0011392120932933

Scott, S., Prior, L., Wood, F., & Gray, J. (2005). Repositioning the patient: The implications of being 'at risk'. *Social Science & Medicine*, *60*(8), 1869–1879. https://doi.org/10.1016/j.socscimed.2004.08.020

Silber, I. F. (2018). Gifts in *Rites of Passage* or gifts as rites of passage? Standing at the threshold between van Gennep and Marcel Mauss. *Journal of Classical Sociology*, *18*(4), 348–360. https://doi.org/10.1177/1468795X18789017

Silver, I. (1996). Role transitions, objects, and identity. *Symbolic Interaction*, *19*(1), 1–20. https://doi.org/10.1525/si.1996.19.1.1

Suárez-Orozco, C., Yoshikawa, H., Teranishi, R. T., & Suárez-Orozco, M. M. (2011). Growing up in the shadows: The developmental implications of unauthorized status. *Harvard Educational Review*, *81*(3), 438–472, 619–620.

Szakolczai, A. (2009). Liminality and experience: Structuring transitory situations and transformative events. *International Political Anthropology*, *2*(1), 141–172.

Szakolczai, A. (2016). Processes of social flourishing and their liminal collapse: Elements to a genealogy of globalization. *The British Journal of Sociology*, *67*(3), 435–455. https://doi.org/10.1111/1468-4446.12213

Szakolczai, A. (2017). Permanent (trickster) liminality: The reasons of the heart and of the mind. *Theory & Psychology, 27*(2), 231–248. https://doi.org/10.1177/0959354317694095

Thomassen, B. (2009). The uses and meaning of liminality. *International Political Anthropology, 2*(1), 5–28.

Thomassen, B. (2012). Émile Durkheim between Gabriel Tarde and Arnold van Gennep: Founding moments of sociology and anthropology. *Social Anthropology, 20*(3), 231–249. https://doi.org/10.1111/j.1469-8676.2012.00204.x

Turner, V. (1967). Betwixt and between: The liminal period in rites de passage. In V. Turner (Ed.), *The forest of symbols: Aspects of Ndembu ritual* (pp. 93–111). Cornell University Press.

Turner, V. (1985). Epilogue: Are there universals of performance in myth, ritual, and drama? In E. Turner (Ed.), *On the edge of the Bush: Anthropology as experience* (pp. 291–301). University of Arizona Press.

Turner, V., & Turner, E. (1978). *Image and pilgrimage in Christian culture: Anthropological perspective*. Columbia University Press.

Turner, V. (1991 [1969]). *The ritual process: Structure and anti-structure*. Cornell University Press.

Wilson, M. (2002). 'I am the prince of pain, for I am a princess in the Brain': Liminal transgender identities, narratives and the elimination of ambiguities. *Sexualities, 5*(4), 425–448. https://doi.org/10.1177/1363460702005004003

Wiltshire, G., Clarke, N. J., Phoenix, C., & Bescoby, C. (2020). Organ transplant recipients' experiences of physical activity: Health, self-care, and transliminality. *Qualitative Health Research, 31*(2), 385–398. https://doi.org/10.1177/1049732320967915

Wimark, T. (2021). Homemaking and perpetual liminality among queer refugees. *Social & Cultural Geography, 22*(5), 647–665. https://doi.org/10.1080/14649365.2019.1619818

van Gennep, A. (1960 [1909]). *The rites of passage* (M. B. Vizedom & G. L. Caffee Trans.). University of Chicago Press.

2 Turning Liminal

As of April 2020, there have been only about 10,000 cumulative infection cases in Korea, a tiny number compared to 34 million cases three years later. However, death rates have been high; hospital beds, protective masks, and hand sanitizers are in short; no vaccines are available, nor any economic relief measures are in place; while social gatherings in any form are prohibited, the infected are being blamed for their misfortune as if they did something wrong. In this situation, the experience of getting infected by coronaviruses is loaded with uncertainties that hardly fall into the existing, clear-cut representations of experience, such as the ill and the healthy. Due to the novelty of these emerging viruses, it remains largely unsettled how to prevent the infection with valid prophylactic measures like vaccines or treat it with effective ex-post interventions. Meanwhile, those at risk of infection and those declared infected have remained suspicious and doubtful about possible infection and recovery at once. Falling outside the conventional clear-cut categories, therefore, the infected have represented the disease as a set of experiences: feeling strange, unusual, mysterious, and nonexistent; feeling incompatible, conflicting, confused, paradoxical, and monstrous while being exposed to two or more categories of experience; and feeling fragile, surrounded by multiple forces and elements in the world.

These ways of turning liminal during the pandemic are thematized summarily in a qualitative coding frame in Figure 2.1. Turning liminal, or falling outside conventional status categories and losing the totality and whole of individuality, manifests in three terms: estrangement, conflicts/paradox, and fragility amid multiplex forces. Estrangement, in turn, becomes evident in two aspects of the self: the personal bodily self and the relational self. Conflicts and paradox are revealed through six sub-themes, such as feeling well but judged sick; a virus-human blend; treatment with no cure; testing dehospitalization after all waits; dehospitalization without a real sense of recovery; and being a risk to others and at risk of being (re-)infected at once. Finally, the infected refer to their fragility as being surrounded by various social forces such as mundane routines,

DOI: 10.4324/9781003493723-3

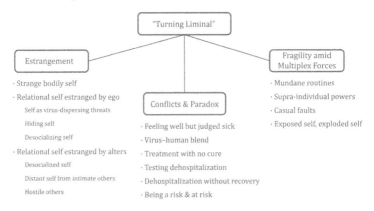

Figure 2.1 Experiential Manifestations of Liminality Due to Infection

supra-individual powers, casual personal faults, and exposure. These are how liminality comes into being lived experiences.

Although the literature implies that people in liminality sometimes feel the natural flow of periods – periodicity and rhythms (van Gennep, 1960 [1909]) – that are constitutive of the totality of life in liminality (Turner & Turner, 1978), this study finds nobody representing their initial infection experience in those terms. Instead, only people who have somehow learned to live with the infection come to reflect on their experience in similar terms retrospectively (see Chapter 4). In the following, pseudonyms are used in parentheses at the end of direct quotes inside double quotation marks.

Estrangement

Strange Bodily Self

Upon developing unusual bodily symptoms around the time when they turn positive on the COVID-19 test, people start feeling strange, mysterious, and unsure about themselves. Although it feels strange and undeniably extant, people do not know for a while what it is exactly. It is interesting that most of the infected have only mild bodily symptoms, except for a few who develop serious symptoms like high fevers and acute muscle pains. The infected are left clueless, therefore, while the conventional categories of experience fail to deliver their lived experience. In those circumstances, people dominantly refer to "the strange bodily self." Italics in the following quotes are the emphatic instances of this strange self. Strangeness is often accompanied by fear and dread (Chang and Wook 2).

I rarely catch a cold. Even when I do, I usually don't have a fever. This time, however, it was *strange* that I had a mild fever. So, I stopped meeting others. … I kept watching over my bodily condition for a week or so. The fever didn't go away. Instead, I started to get other symptoms additionally. I had difficulty in breathing and felt pain while breathing. Then, I realized that I was not able to smell or taste things. I even attempted to smell naphthalene balls at my nose, but I smelled nothing. At that moment, I knew that *something was wrong* with me.

(Wook 1)

Ever since my friends and I had visited a wine bar together, we *strangely* took turns feeling down. My old-time sinusitis got worse. A friend took cold remedies. Although we didn't know at the time whether it was Covid-19, we told one another that it *didn't feel alright* and there was *something*. … Another friend simply didn't smell nor taste, without any cold-like symptoms. We were *not sure* what it was.

(Han 1)

(While sitting at the table with family,) fish was burning on the grill behind me. However, I wasn't smelling anything. I didn't taste anything. I had meat, knowing it was only because of its texture inside the mouth. I kept thinking '*it is strange*' for quite a while.

(Han 2)

It was *mysterious* that I didn't smell things. At first, I didn't know I couldn't smell things. When I suddenly came to know it, I talked to the doctor who nonetheless was *not sure* whether it was from Covid-19. I spent one month living like that without knowing that the smell loss was from the infection.

(Hee)

I was utterly *suspicious*. Two days after I joined my friends at a bar, I kept having symptoms that people now say are Covid-19-related. In addition, all my friends had cold-like symptoms at the same time. Being troubled, I went to the doctor only to hear that it wasn't the infection. However, I wasn't feeling well. I was *caught between suspicion and doubt* for some time. Before seeing the doctor, I hoped it was Covid-19. After hearing from the doctor that it was not it, though, I wasn't fully sure that I was free of it; I *doubted* the doctor and kept *suspecting* Covid-19. ... I kept wearing the face-mask. I locked myself inside my room at home and had meals alone.

(Gan)

I felt stressed out. I had only a mild fever for a couple days. I didn't get anything concrete and persuasive from the hospital that I was infected with the virus. Yet I was told that I was infected. *I couldn't believe that I was infected nor that I was free from the virus. I couldn't trust myself.*

(Min)

I was scared that I might never recover from the infection. (As a nurse,) I knew how medical interventions proceed through diagnosis, prognosis, and gradual measures of improvement. However, *I didn't hear any clear diagnosis or step-by-step plans* to recover from the illness. Interventions were simply full of *conjectures*. People took conjectures as professional interventions.

(Chang)

Things that I had not experienced happened to me. I suddenly realized that it was so scary to have no smell or taste. It was utterly *dread-ful* because I suspected that I might never get back those senses. Without senses, eating is no more eating. ... While I was watching people on the next (hospital) beds in serious conditions, I came to realize that people could die easily. And I was going through pains that I had never experienced before. This made me scared because *I had never known those pains before. I feared myself.* While having a high fever and feeling like fainting in pain, I suspected myself if I was dying. *So, I thought about writing a will one moment; on the next moment, however, my thinking suddenly faded into the struggle with bodily pains.*

(Wook 2)

Relational Self Estranged by the Ego

The initial strangeness often extends to further estrangement that the ego initiates regarding the self and others. The following descriptions demonstrate that the damage that the infection has incurred on the ego is mostly social-relational. To the extent to which the self is composed of the relational self as well as the personal self, these social-relational damages have impacts on how people feel about themselves.

The following first set of quotes highlights that the infected people estrange themselves by perceiving themselves as virus-dispersing threats or viruses per se in relation to distant and close others. This perception pervades the infected not only when they get initially infected but also when they are discharged from the hospital without being assured of their recovery. This self-perception results in people's voluntary disclosure of private information like credit card uses and personal whereabouts around the suspected time of infection, sometimes to the point of "ridicule" (Sun). These responses resonate with public authorities' efforts for comprehensive contact tracing.

> *I didn't think I was a victim. Instead, I was extremely worried that I might bring harm to others.* Rather than taking my infection as unrighteous and unfair, I feared that others might be infected by me. If I had infected others, I would've had to blame myself. This self-blame was what I feared most. … I voluntarily told everything to the health authority about the places I had visited and at what time in order to inform others of the possible dangerous contact with me. … In public transit to and from work (after the hospital discharge), I wouldn't face other passengers but turned my face away or looked down. At work, I did the same when others came to me in the hallway. It was a kind of new me. That is because *I felt like I still had viruses inside me.* The treatment experience seemed to affect this. *While being treated in the hospital, the repeated virus test results had swung between negative and positive unpredictably.* I didn't worry too much about me being re-infected but cared about infecting others, especially older people. I used to work at the intensive care unit (ICU) and saw many old people pass away with pneumonia in the end.
>
> (Chang)

> It seems ridiculous now, but (when I discovered I was infected), *I was obsessed with reporting (to the health authority) all my whereabouts with exact times.* So, I ran through all my credit card bills and receipts to report the places and times of my movements.
>
> (Sun)

> I live in a town well known for strawberry farming. (It was a peak time for strawberry harvest when I was infected.) The farmers were put in a difficult situation because there was a rumor that market distributors wouldn't collect the strawberries from my town *for fear of the Covid-19 viruses from me and my family.*
>
> (Song)

> I used to be pretty outgoing. But, upon my infection and hospital discharge, I found myself stuck at home. I felt afraid. … My workplace was changing due to me. People used to be lenient about the

facemask. But suddenly, they all started wearing it. When I stepped into the office, they *put on the masks. Without me, they often didn't. It hurt me a little.* ... Many things were murky. People were saying that *I might get positive again because the viruses hadn't really gone away, and they could resurface in me any time.* ... I wasn't sure either. When I felt a fever on my face, I immediately took the temperature and felt troubled.

(Gan)

When I returned from abroad, I didn't have a fever or other suspicious symptoms on the entry check. So, I was allowed by the government to go straight home. But, *I didn't go home or meet my family* because I was worried that I might infect my sister, who is a nurse, and another family member, who is a doctor. People recommended that I'd better not contact medical professionals in the family because they were extremely wanted and needed to be protected for the public. I stayed at a hotel for some time.

(Bae)

My family did it in a strict way because mom was working for the city government. Upon seeing me returning from the UK to the airport, mom asked me *to cover up with a raincoat for fear that I might infect her and Dad* and stopped Dad, who insisted on talking to me, from talking to me in the car all the way home. At home, I secluded myself in my room.

(Seul)

I learned it was awfully stressful to worry that I might've infected my family. ... I was taking job-related courses in the UK and was living with a local family in London before I got on the plane back home to Korea due to border shutdowns. ... While not knowing the result of my infection test yet, I had dinner with my husband right after I got home and enjoyed being relieved to meet him after a while abroad away from home. Within the next 24 hours, I got hospitalized. *It made me so worried that I might've infected him.* ... *I shouldn't have dined with him. I regretted it repeatedly for two weeks. It was horrible.* When I finally learned that he was alright, *I thought it was lucky that it was only me.* ... Then, I called the local couple in the UK with whom I had lived and said I was infected and asked them to take tests. They had been so nice to me that I didn't want to be the one who infected them and got them in trouble. ... *I kept worrying. What if I infected my friends, my family, or my husband?*

(Ree)

When I tested positive, I was living with Mom, an older sister, her husband, and their kids. So, all of them had to take the tests because of me. Luckily, they all tested negative. However, until we finally learned it and were relieved of infection worries, I had to go through many difficulties. Since I had no symptoms, I was sleeping with my old Mom, aged over 70, who has some health problems. I was having meals with all the family until I got notified that I was positive. One of the nephews was a senior in high school preparing for the college exam and, nevertheless, was not able to go to school out of concern about infection. My sister and brother-in-law had to stop working for a while. *It was all because of me. I felt really, really sorry for the family.* I hoped nobody ever needed to go through it like I did. ... We don't have to go through it. *It is not like I can be sick all by myself. Infection affects the whole family.* If I had infected any of them, it would've been so heartbreaking and bitter.

(Jin)

While I was in the hospital, I talked to my mom on the phone almost every day and heard that the city government asked the whole family to stay home. The government delivered home a box of emergency food each day. The family was grounded. *I felt guilty to them.*

(Han)

The following set of quotes shows that, as a result, the infected shut themselves from others by hiding part of the true self and not sharing the deep-seated worries and emotional hardships arising from the infection experiences. It is ironic and agonizing that people hide themselves away from others in fear of losing and in pursuit of keeping their precious social ties to those others (Sook, Seul, and Min). Sometimes, people intend to secure the self by hiding if they are solitary and disconnected from others permanently (Cheol). The hiding is not only from distant others but also from close family. In these manners, hideaways amount to a surprising situation where it is difficult for an infected person to know another infected one (Hee). Each of the infected is left all alone.

Upon testing positive after returning from abroad, I was caught by great fear, especially the fear that I would be isolated from others. ... I was so scared that *I hid the fact that I was infected and, instead, replied to others that I was in a precautionary quarantine at home and pretended to be O.K.* ... I knew that people were criticizing the infected like me for being infected by having carelessly made a trip, in my case, to attend a daughter's wedding in a dangerous foreign country. *I was so scared of losing my shared life with those others.*

(Sook)

I didn't and still don't know how I got infected. If I had known where and when, it would've been a lot easier to talk to people who had been in close contact with me. The friends I had hung out with in the UK wondered where I got infected. They suspected it was in the airplane heading back to Korea rather than during the time when I had been with them in the UK. *In that suspicion, I sensed their wish that they hadn't been with me who might've already gotten infected. It was difficult not to be able to say exactly where I think I got it while I knew this wish.*

(Seul)

I was even worried how my close friends would react to me if I told them what happened to me and my mom. *I feared that they would turn hostile to me.* ... Even after de-hospitalization, routine life was impossible. *I felt very uneasy about meeting friends. So, I rarely left home and got stuck in my room.*

(Min)

Some neighbors made a fuss and raided the management office, requesting endless disinfections around my apartment unit which had been empty since all family were admitted to hospitals. They treated my place like that of a sex perpetrator. Once going through these, *I never felt like opening up my infection story to others* except a few.

(Cheol)

Close people knew that I was infected and cared about my health. But *I doubted that others would sympathize with me much. So, I didn't let them know* of my condition ... People treated the infection as a loathsome disease.

(Jin)

A mother of a friend of my kid told me that she was happy to see me released healthy from the infection treatment. I was surprised because *I had not told* any mom of my daughter's friends. On second thought, *I felt thankful to them because they had pretended not to know of my infection and treated me the same.* Only after the hospital discharge they sent their regards to me. ... *Isn't it interesting that it is so difficult to meet in person someone infected with the virus while the government says that more people are being infected? It was really hard to find anyone infected near me.* It is the same now. It seems that the infected people are *hiding themselves.* It's only my suspicion.

(Hee)

Even when they are released from facilities, therefore, the infected literally do not socialize with others, like family, friends, and coworkers

(Sun, Chang, Dong, Kwang 1, Bae, Sook 1, Sung, Gan, and Ree 1), to the extent that loneliness surpasses infection worries (Kwang 1, Ree 1, and Min). When they talk to others, they willingly do not deliver their personal experiences of how they got infected and treated in medical facilities (Min, Cheol 1, Kwang 2, Sook 2, Han, Ree 2, Cheol 2, and Hee). In doing so, they often find themselves losing self-confidence (Sung) and personal integrity (Hee). Intentional desocialization takes place at work, school, home, streets, jogging courses, and public transportation.

> I felt that I would be infected again and hospitalized any time. So, for one week or so after hospital discharge, *I brought home lunch with me and had it alone in my office. I didn't hang out with coworkers for lunch* at the company cafeteria. … *After work, I came straight home* without stopping by other places. It was like simply home, work, home, work, repeatedly. … *It was traumatic.* I couldn't go to restaurants or places where people flocked.
>
> (Sun)

> Honestly, I would've been just like those people distancing the once infected unless I had been mature and considerate. So, I understood them. But *I couldn't help but drop my head down in front of others even though I told myself it was alright. I wasn't able to blend into coworkers for lunch.* … I got nervous and sweated when I was with many others.
>
> (Chang)

> After returning to work, I took *home lunch* to work. The other coworkers who had not been infected yet did so as well. Before I became infected, we used to have lunch together at cafes and restaurants. I felt sorry and responsible for all this.
>
> (Dong)

> I literally *didn't meet any person for almost two months* after discharge. … It was half voluntary and half compulsory. … It was so difficult. So, at a certain point, I couldn't bear it anymore, and I really wanted to meet people no matter what. … *Loneliness became greater than infection worries. Loneliness devoured infection worries.* It was a sad story.
>
> (Kwang 1)

> There was news on the possibility that people who recovered might still carry viruses. … I didn't go home from hospital but to a hotel. *I voluntarily put myself in seclusion for two more weeks.*
>
> (Bae)

Once getting home dismissed from the hospital, *I didn't leave home for two or three months. I didn't go to work.* I told my boss about my fear. Whenever I had a headache or muscle ache, I kept taking corona tests. ... I didn't get out of my apartment except when I dumped trash. For trash runs, I covered up myself with a mask and gloves. *It was fearful* to go outside.

(Sook 1)

When I resumed my work, I couldn't look at others in the eyes. *I wasn't able to hold up my face before others. Although I was a teacher, I didn't look at students in their eyes. Because I felt like a sinner.* ... It was for about a month. ... I lived like a sinner. ... As a teacher, *I couldn't advise the kids on anything.* I couldn't tell them to get orderly at the school cafeteria because *I was blaming myself* for not having abided by the precautionary recommendations against Covid-19. *I lost confidence* in front of the kids, about my life, and in front of others. Then, support from close people helped me to overcome it.

(Sung)

I didn't share plates and bowls with my family. For two weeks, *I stayed all alone even at home.* My parents had wanted to go to a motel.

(Gan)

I was so worried that I told my husband not to come to the room where *I kept myself away* from him until I would get cleared on a follow-up infection test. But he insisted that it was okay to get infected from me. ... He said it was impossible to live without seeing each other. So, he dropped in the room from time to time or *stood at the door, and we greeted afar.*

(Ree 1)

Even after de-hospitalization, routine life was impossible. *I felt very uneasy about meeting friends.* So, I rarely left home and got stuck in my room. ... Seeing how people reacted to the infected people, *I thought it impossible to live in this country* once people knew about my infection. ... It was a totally different life. *I cried every day due to loneliness.* I had to go for outdoor exercise at dawn when there were not many people. I didn't go for groceries but ordered them home. *I locked myself up.*

(Min)

After hospital discharge, *my wife and I hated meeting neighbors.* So, we kind of fled overnight and hit the road to a pension in a remote area, a cabin in the woods, a motel at the seashore, and others. *We chose to disappear from our neighborhood* for some time.

(Cheol 1)

One day, there was an on-campus academic conference about Covid-19. During presentations and discussions, my advising professor blurted out, 'Kwang had a very close experience with Covid-19. What do you think, Kwang?' I (a graduate student) was not able to say that I was upset at his spotting me there. I was at a loss for what to say. There were many people who I hadn't seen in the past half a year, and *most didn't know that I had been infected with Covid-19*. It was so sudden that I was extremely perplexed. … *I was so embarrassed that I couldn't look around to see how others were reacting. … I had wanted my infection to be forgotten by people and to live unnoticed.*

(Kwang 2)

Since I was hospitalized for a long time, I went to the insurance company to get reimbursed for any relevant costs. But *the words, 'I had been infected with Covid-19,' didn't come out of my mouth*, when the agent asked me what my hospitalization was for. Instead, I said that I would come back later, and I took off.

(Sook 2)

When I was discharged from hospital, not many were infected across the country. *A simple utterance of 'corona' would startle and freeze people. So, I didn't tell anybody but close friends* about my infection.

(Han)

I wasn't able to talk about my infection. Most people didn't know about it. I informed only about ten people. The infection story was *a kind of secret*. … I never told coworkers or friends who were close to coworkers. … Then, (after the plasma donation), I felt proud of myself. I felt like talking about it to others around me, but I couldn't. I felt great for several days *all by myself*. … I unwittingly talked to a coworker about my infection. She sort of found fault in me, saying how I could not tell her. I was baffled. If she had been a person who really cared about me, she would've first asked whether I was ok. But her first reaction wasn't that. I came to realize that she was distant to me.

(Ree 2)

When I needed a haircut, *I couldn't manage to go to the shop that I frequent. I felt uneasy about getting the service without letting them know of my situation.* I didn't want to let them know, but I needed a haircut.

I went to a shop in another city on my business trip there. The designer asked me to take off the mask, but I didn't. She said I was overly careful (of being infected by others). Even so, *I didn't tell* that I had already been infected.

(Cheol 2)

I didn't talk about my infection to others very much because I worried that they might develop prejudice against me. Although I didn't intend to hide it, *this kind of withholding made me feel like I was not an honest person.* It was difficult.

(Hee)

Relational Self Estranged by Alters

Those three instances of self-estrangement often mirror alter-initiated alienation. Even when the infected do not isolate themselves from others, furthermore, they frequently feel that others distance themselves from the infected. Alter-driven estrangement takes three forms. First, people literally do not want to hand out with the once infected. Second, even close and intimate others, like family, friends, and neighbors, distance the infected in unpredicted and yet straightforward manners, such as physical distancing, surveillance, suspicion, doubt, distrust, betrayal, threats, mistreatments, and misrecognition (Song 1, Jin, Seul, Woo, Cheol 1, Hee 1, Min, and Dong 1).

I headed straight home from the airport. *My parents had already blocked the room door and sealed it with vinyl.* I climbed into the room through the window. Then, when I got the positive test result, I climbed out through the window to an ambulance. *My parents completely sealed me off the whole time.* However, they had to be quarantined at home for another two weeks due to my infection. They lived in a stand-alone house in a rural area (Iksan). After boring days of detention, they came outside to the vegetable garden to pluck spinach next to the porch. *A neighbor about 1 km away spotted them and called the health authority to report that the dangerous couple were on the loose.*

(Song 1)

My sister (whose family I was living with) and other siblings (who were not living with me) got really angry at me being infected. Especially my sister did. I was upset at her being like that. But her situation was understandable. She was living with my mom and her kids, one of whom was about to take the college entrance exam. She is also a let-it-explode-first kind of person. So, the whole household tumbled upside down because of me. … While living with me, she seemed to have *cold reactions* from others more than I did. She said one day that *she came to tell who was really close to her and who was not.*

(Jin)

When I was taking language courses in the UK, most classmates went easy on Covid-19 except one from France. She left the classroom whenever someone sneezed in class. She was very sensitive to her surroundings. She was one of my *close friends*. When I came back to Korea and let her know that I got infected, *she took it very seriously, panicked, and ultimately called an ambulance for herself because she was worried that I might've infected her* while we were taking classes together. *I felt as if I had been indebted to her.*

(Seul)

Touchy friends wouldn't see me, even though I persuaded them that I was fully recovered and finally set free from hospital. 'In another three weeks,' they said. I didn't expect it, although it was understandable. Though, it hurt me. It was a good experience.

(Woo)

Some *neighbors* made a fuss and raided the management office, requesting endless disinfections around my apartment unit. ... *They treated my place like that of a sex perpetrator. ... We got a lot (of bad reactions) from neighbors.* When I was in the hospital, they called me and complained about all different things. At that time, my son was discharged from the hospital before me, and he was staying home. My neighbors called and urged me over and again to tell my son to stay put at home, even though he didn't get out of the apartment for weeks. People alleged that they saw him in the elevator without wearing a mask. To defend him, I had to show them the surveillance recordings at the front door. ... *As neighbors distrusted one another, I received a lot of doubts and suspicions from them. ... They didn't believe what I said.*

(Cheol 1)

When my infection case was publicized through the local mom cafe (an online chat room), residents of my apartment complex overwhelmed the management office and requested the exact apartment building, if not the unit number. *The manager in charge exposed the building number.* I felt aggravated and objected to the manager. ... The restaurant where I did part-time work when I got infected suffered real damage. *Many customers called in and poured out abusive words, threatening that it should be closed.*

(Hee 1)

When I read how people reacted to the news reports of my infection and mom's infection, I got extremely angry, and it felt utterly unrighteous. Although it was already sad to be infected, others made it even worse by *mistreating my mom who lived in Daegu (which was famous for the Christian cult Sincheonji that was criticized for generating an enormous number of infection cases during its mystic worship services in crammed places) as the cult member.* She was not. She only got infected by her colleague at work who was a member of the cult. So, I hated those people. *I was even worried about how my close friends would react* to me if I told them what happened to me and my mom. ... When I had a chance to visit my hometown Daegu, I informed old friends of my infection and hospital discharge. *I called for a reunion (in a chat room). All were silent.* Then, I realized that they felt uncomfortable about seeing me. Only after a while they replied that it seemed too early to gather together (although it was one month after my hospital discharge). *I was shocked. Although it's getting weaker, that feeling is still with me* whenever I see those friends.

(Min)

Upon infection, I suffered physically. It lasted only for a couple days. It wasn't that bad. *I was scared the most about the chances* that I might bring harm to others and *others might develop bad impressions of me,* like 'I am a reckless person.' ... My company managers took my infection as damaging the company's reputation when it was publicized where I worked. They seemed to have several phone calls from the press regarding me, and they made public statements on account of me. *They complained to me about this unnecessary extra work.* In the process, *the company made me report what I had done off duty* around the time when I may have contracted the virus. It seemed that *my company took me as a reckless employee.*

(Dong 1)

Third, remote and unknown others who used to be largely indifferent, disinterested, and casual to the ego – i.e., strangers – suddenly turn hostile and concerned with the ego – i.e., challengers and enemies – by developing curiosities, raising questions and doubts, spreading rumors and misinformation, scapegoating, and criminalizing (Cheol 2, Gan, Dong 2, Han, and Kwang). Most often, strangers on the internet (Sung, Song 2, and Hee 2) turn infuriated and antagonistic toward the ego, whom they have little acquaintance with or have false information about, in contrast to those who have known the infected in person and endured them through it all (Kwang and Sung). Interviewees seem to have attempted to ignore those strangers and their reactions, but they often fail to (Cheol 2). These stories embrace the contemporary relevance of Simmel's treatment of the stranger (Simmel, 1908) as a general form of existence or relation that is yet laden with tensions. Under tensions, the stranger as a representative social category refers to the unity of two different things, which can tilt not necessarily to either side. In the pandemic context, it has tilted to the enemy, which necessarily embroils people's heretofore relationship with the stranger. This tilting of the stranger constitutes a third aspect of estrangement.

I didn't really care about those who, for no reason, troubled me. For other instances than the coronavirus infection, they would've troubled me anyway. So, I didn't care. But they were there, indeed. *These people were so concerned with things that had nothing to do with them that they spread on the SNS, like mom cafes, the unsupported rumors regarding my family.* They simply babbled around on things that *they used to be indifferent to and knew nothing about. They suddenly made hostile remarks on us.* I didn't and don't mean to take those people seriously and fight with them, even though they hurt my feelings. They were still strangers to me. *I kept them as strangers but not enemies,* although *they seemed to decide to become enemies rather than strangers to me. ...* But it is different for people who are close to me. Not really a friend, but someone I felt close to made fun of me being hospitalized, saying that my family and I were using up the tax money that he paid. I am rather hot-tempered. I would've slapped him in the face if in person. ... After I was discharged, he made another joke in the chat room (Kakao Talk), saying how come it was only me but not others who got infected. He implied my infection was intentional. I cut him off the contact list in my phone.

(Cheol 2)

I didn't want to read them (online posts) because I knew that I was being criticized for the infection. But my friends bothered to send me the screenshots of what people said online. There were so many untrue stories about me. ... *People posted false information while pretending that they had known me well. It was egregious. ... It was scary when the information was true.* People posted details about me: how old I was, where I lived, where I usually went, and who my friends were. It's so scary. I admit that I wasn't considerate enough not to go to the wine bar. But *facing all the twisted information about myself and feeling threatened by strangers was too much. ...* I was having unnecessary *criticism of my life from strangers. ... We were scapegoats.* There were not many infection cases then, and we were only the 6th and 7th cases. Until then, the other cases were from honeymoon trips and international travel. *People didn't know where to pour out their frustrations in front of the infectious disease.* Then, we were there as reckless wine bar-goers. *To them, wine bars were unjustifiable, unlike honey-moon trips (for young girls).*

(Gan)

People started talking about me on the internet. I was described as someone who was cheating on my partner. *I suddenly became famous as a cheating man.* ... At work, *many people (who used to be indifferent to me) became attracted to me.* They were careful but *inquisitive* about my personal life. ... My girlfriend went to a friend's wedding and heard strangers talking about her without knowing that she was standing next to them. ... Others didn't care whether it was true, but they seemed faithful to believe the rumor. That was unbelievable. ... Once being infected, *I was treated as an evildoer* in the internet news and people's replies to them. ... *I was only an unlucky man before this infectious disease, but these reactions stigmatized me as a wrongdoer.* It hurt the feeling. ... I thought it was unfair. *This disease was not caused by the church. The disease simply befell a greater-than-usual number of people at once during the church events. But the press described it as if the church had caused the problem.* This image ran counter to the idea that the church should be an institute delivering love and care (and not harm) to neighbors. I felt sorrowful for this unfounded and manufactured conflict. We (believers) had simply gathered for worship in accordance with common sense at that time. There had been no one infected in Busan, and the press had promoted that citizens should continue running the economy without being unnecessarily intimidated by the virus. But, once it broke out, all the responsibility fell upon us. *The church-wide infection happened opportunistically; people thought it happened out of selfish misjudgment.* ... People made fictitious stories, although things happened during the routine daily life like commuting, eat-outs, and worship. *Things simply had happened by chance. But bystanders made hasty, ready judgments; they talked about the infected without reservation; the online press circulated untrue stories and conjectures.*

(Dong 2)

News about us were all over the place. ... We used to go to wine bars. But *it suddenly turned out to be something evil in others' eyes, especially in the online mom cafe.* They rebuked, 'Wine bars at this moment?' So, we thought it was our fault to go there.

(Han)

I felt helpless. I couldn't do anything, although *I wanted to protest that I hadn't committed a crime. I was simply a weak person, and I got infected more easily. That's who I am. Most people around me knew it. But the news reports and online posts* treated me like a criminal. ... My body is susceptible to infectious diseases more than others. I had already been infected with the Avian Flu in 2010. So, I had always remained alert whenever there was a nationwide advisory against infectious diseases. But I got infected once more this time. *I was already personally dejected, and the ill-informed news reports made it worse.*

(Kwang)

I realized that people would rather criticize others than hope to know what exactly happened to them. *Since it's anonymous on the internet, and when the infected were strangers, people tended to turn aggressive and fault-finding easily. If they had known me and I had known them, they would've been more watchful* for fear of harm backfiring to them. People were simple-mindedly busy speaking lowly for strangers who went through what they hadn't.

(Sung)

I am okay now, but I was going through a hard time then. ... I was reading what *others replied to the internet news about my case. There were many swears and curses that are unspeakable,* like 'you should've died abroad (the US),' 'why did you come back?' and 'if you bring any harm to my parents who are living in the same area as you, I'd kill you.'

(Song 2)

While in hospital, I got cuts in my heart from the online posts about me. I didn't get infected because I did something wrong. But people kept criticizing me, *putting me in big fear (of others who I shouldn't have dreaded).* So, I kept hiding away; I was heartbroken and depressed. ... It was so rare an occasion to meet someone infected because I hadn't told people about my infection. Then, I once met someone whose parents got infected. I heard that they suffered a lot. Then, *I found myself wondering and so inquisitive about how on earth they got infected. 'Are they believers in a religious cult like Sincheonji?' 'Did they not follow the precautionary measures against it?' I was judging them, although I was being hurt by others who judged me.* I myself was holding that horrible prejudice. I got scared of the press releases (that had erroneously produced all these).

(Hee 2)

Conflicts and Paradox

Feeling Well but Judged Sick

Many interviewees have experienced conflicts and mismatches between their subjective judgments of themselves and the objective test results by the health authority. It is more demanding to make sense of subjective and objective realities that do not agree with one another than it is challenging to know how subjective reality becomes objective reality (Berger & Luckmann, 1991 [1967]). The following occasions of "(subjectively) feeling well but (objectively) judged sick" lead not only to producing hesitancy and doubt about either subjective self-knowledge or the authoritative science (Hwan, Seul, and Han) but also to amplifying people's worry, fear, and psychological distress about the seemingly unintelligible viruses that produce these conflicts and mismatches (Han, Gan, Min, Jin, and Cheol). The viruses are so threatening as they are unknowable in producing conflicting experiences.

> I was *an asymptomatic infection* case. I hadn't realized anything unusual about me until I got notified of the test result. Then, the treatment process kicked in. … *It made no sense.* I had never doubted that I was okay. If there had been some symptoms, I could've been ready to accept the test result. *I was stupefied. It was unreal.*
>
> (Hwan)

> *I didn't know what to say to nurses and doctors* once I was hospitalized according to the test result. When they asked me about symptoms, *I was so free of symptoms. It was so embarrassing.*
>
> (Seul)

> I wasn't feeling well. I took cold medicines, mostly stayed home, and didn't meet others. I didn't eat with my family and wore a mask at home just in case. *About two weeks had passed that way, and I got over most of the bodily symptoms.* Then, the news broke out that the wine bar owner got infected, whom I had visited with my friends around the time when I started feeling sluggish. *My friends and I were all shocked* and called on one another to take the test. *We all got positive (with no bodily symptoms)*, and ambulances took us away. … As soon as I heard about the news of the bar owner, I thought about me possibly getting infected as well, *but I persistently doubted it.* All the while, I got really scared. *I got scared* not because I had bodily sufferings but *because I might've infected others while not having known it all.*
>
> (Han)

> I thought it was a common cold. I took cold medicine and got better. *I was about to get it over as a cold. Then, I was notified that I was infected.* I had no physical suffering. But it was mostly mental problems. *I became extremely sensitive and vulnerable, mentally.*
>
> (Gan)

I had *no symptoms*. Yet I was *locked up* in the hospital. It was very *stress-ful. … I didn't sleep well in hospital. I couldn't breathe well.* Doctors said it was all mental and had nothing to do with the infection. … On the other hand, *I felt so sorry for taking up a heavy-equipped hospital room all by myself.* So, as soon as they offered a transfer to a community treatment center, I immediately agreed.

(Min)

I was admitted to a community treatment center. … *The disease was uncertain in many ways.* People didn't know much about the disease. The government didn't have any systematic procedure to address it. Although admitted to a government facility, I felt great fear. *I knew I was okay and had no symptoms, but they said I was infected. This (mismatch) caused a lot of psychological burden to me. I felt okay, but they said I was sick and infected.* … At first, *I didn't believe the positive test result* from a primary care center because I had no symptoms.

(Jin)

I had a mild fever and a sore throat for a few days, which disappeared with painkillers. After that, *I had no symptoms but remained hospital-ized for one month and ten days.* … The infection notice and hospi-talization happened so quickly that I was stunned. It was stressful … because the news reports about it seemed like an exaggeration. It was overly nerve-racking and agitating. It was more than raising people's prudent awareness of the disease. The press should've been more care-ful. *It simply scared people by saying that people in the 60s and more would die of the disease with no exception. … I myself felt alright. But my old-aged friends were overwhelmed with worries about me. They didn't believe that I was okay. They thought I was lying to relieve them. It was not easy to deal with their reactions (and how I actually felt about my health at the same time).*

(Cheol)

The Virus–Human Blend

Another source of conflict and paradox is identified among the interview-ees who see themselves as human beings annexed to the coronaviruses. This virus–human experience has several colors. It develops into self-doubt (Min) and the confused perception of the self as a pitiful zombie or plague (Sook and Woo). The blend and complex are simply monstrous, given people's reluctance to accept the reality where uncontrollable det-rimental viruses besiege people. When one reconciles with one's uneasy self-perception of the human–virus complex, it is not always guaranteed that distant others would come to terms with this reconciliation. For example, Kwang and Hee identify themselves with the viruses. However, they report that it is difficult for others to be open to this identification. Instead, remote others criminalize – instead of normalizing – the human–virus experience (Kwang); they embrace the infected ego but distance the virus inside the ego, which produces unusual agony to the ego who sees the virus as part of the self if reluctantly (Hee).

> Even after the hospital discharge, *I couldn't believe myself. I felt like I still had the viruses inside me.* There were so many rumors about the viruses. … I had long awaited the discharge. *Once I got released, though, it was not the end but another beginning (of confusion). I couldn't believe myself.*
>
> (Min)

> I could bear with the separation for treatment and the mild bodily suffering. But I couldn't put up with my worries about how others would think of me. When I had seen the news of the infected on TV, I had often had pity on them and distanced them as if they'd been zombies. Then, this thing happened to me. *I had to fear that others would look at me like a disagreeable zombie.*
>
> (Sook)

> When I was at the treatment center, *nurses were very watchful around me because I was carrying the viruses.* When I reached out to get the meal tray because I felt sorry for their every service, they told me not to move and insisted they would do everything for me. So, I didn't move an inch. They cleaned it all when the mealtime was over. *It hurt my feelings because they treated me like an untouchable person with the plague. It hurt me deeply sometimes.*
>
> (Woo)

> I felt helpless. I couldn't do anything, although I wanted to protest that I hadn't committed a crime. I was simply a weak person, and I got infected more easily. *That's who I am. I'm prone to viruses and infections.* Most people around me knew it. But the news reports and online posts *treated me like a criminal.* … My body is susceptible to infectious diseases more than others.
>
> (Kwang)

> My whole family tested negative. I didn't infect anyone. All I went to was to a grocery store. I didn't harm anyone. *Nevertheless, I was hurt a lot* when I was reading online posts. *These posts were not about me, though. They were directed to the viruses, the Covid-19 disease, and other infected people. But I felt that these assaults and criticisms in the posts*

*were targeting me. The criticism and distancing toward the viruses felt
like those toward me. ... as the host of viruses ...*

(Hee)

Treatment with No Cure

Once admitted to a hospital or a community treatment center, which is
not determined only by the severity of symptoms but the availability of
these facilities, the infected face a paradoxical situation in which they get
forcibly detained in a facility and yet do not get real cures because there
is no cure yet. The paradox of being hospitalized without being properly
treated is revealed in several forms, while everyone acknowledges that
this paradox is inevitable. These paradoxical experiences make people re-
calibrate what it means to be institutionalized and what it means to be
treated for medical conditions like infection. People realize that institutional admission and treatment do not necessarily presume the clear-cut
definitions of the sick nor promise to restore the unequivocal status of
the healthy in the future. This vague situation troubles people with more
worries and fears about the infectious disease (Chang, Gan, Bae, and
Han). Subsequently, some people cling even more to whatever medical
professionals do, even if all they do is symptomatic treatments (Dong and
Kwang). Some of these people even become active participants in clinical
trials in the hope of a real cure (Hwan). Conversely, others occasionally
become resigned (Ree, Song, and Jin) and reject the symptomatic treatments at once (Cheol).

> *I was scared that I might never recover from the infection.* I knew how
> medical interventions proceed through diagnosis, prognosis, and
> gradual measures of health recovery. However, *I didn't hear any clear
> diagnosis or step-by-step plans to recover from the illness. Interventions
> were simply full of conjectures. People took conjectures as treatments.
> Knowing all this, I was more scared than others.*
>
> (Chang)

> *There was no promise or prediction* about how and when these treat-
> ments would end. Little information was available. *This made worries
> greater.* ... The low and continuous *machine sound in the negative
> pressure room (isolation room) got on my nerves. It magnified the fear
> (of being isolated with no cure for infection).*
>
> (Gan)

> Sometimes *I felt like we were part of medical experiments.* I honestly
> still don't know whether any drugs were ever effective.
>
> (Bae)

Diagnoses were made on the phone within the facility. I heard I got early-stage pneumonia. The doctor asked me if I would take anti-viral drugs for *symptomatic treatment*, and I conceded. I took them for 4 to 5 days and *suffered a lot of adverse effects*. I had a nausea and felt like vomiting. The doctor had told me that I could stop the drugs if I started not seeing well. So, I kept checking my eyesight to see if I was seeing distant things well, and I felt alright until days after I finished the pills. I felt like I didn't see well and thought something was wrong with one of my eyes. *I rushed to report it to the doctor.* He said that it was unusual to undergo a vision problem within that short amount of time from the pills and to have a problem with only one eye, and *tried to relieve me. However, I remained scared and suspicious.* Eye doctors (other than the infection-related workers) were not available in the facility, *making me more nervous.* ... Looking back, *I don't think it was necessary* to stay confined within a facility for so long. *There was no cure, and I was simply kept in quarantine while being put on cold medicines.* I am thankful for all the meals prepared for me. But it was too long.

(Han)

There were *no vaccines and no cures*. Instead, I took the AIDS drug Kaletra, which I would've never had. Honestly, the drug was scary. *'Is it okay for me to take it? Isn't it harming my body?' I kept suspecting.* ... There were many mysteries about the symptomatic treatments using the drug. People talked about different adverse effects online. One professor talked about something called brain fog, which means you can't think clearly. Others talked about the lung changing into fibers. So, *I was worried that I might develop these adverse effects on me and live with them forever.* ... *But I didn't tell the healthcare workers that I wouldn't take the drug. That's because I wanted to get over the infection in any way, easy or difficult. I had to do something.* I couldn't let it go without trying anything for fear of adverse effects. *Without a second thought, I took the drug and suffered adverse effects like diarrhea and skin troubles.*

(Dong)

I took the malaria drug Hydroxychloroquine. Although we now know it doesn't work, doctors and I didn't know it then, and we tried it because there were no other ways. *It was symptomatic therapy.* ... The healthcare workers had never faced the disease before. All they could do was *try every possible measure, like CT, MRI, X-rays, morning pills (if not a cure), evening pills, three meals a day, etc. They did their best. But we were never relieved.* ... I saw they did everything they could. They just didn't know the cure. ... I thought that the symptomatic treatment with the AIDS and malaria drugs was *better than nothing. The fear for the coronavirus was way greater than the fear for these untested drugs.*

(Kwang)

There was *no treatment other than vital sign checks.* Usually, they ran X-rays on my lung and gave out pills for headaches. There was *no cure.* ... Doctors used some alternative drugs originally for malaria and AIDS. ... My doctor gave me an AIDS medication (Kaletra) and said that, although he wasn't sure, the AIDS drug seemed to be more effective in *controlling the symptoms* than malaria drugs. So, although I was suffering from the adverse effects of the drug, I didn't switch to a malaria drug, which was believed to have fewer adverse effects. *I was concerned about adverse effects, but I wanted any drugs that would make the suffering (from Covid-19) disappear more quickly, even if they were not real cures. I kept on the AIDS drug. ... Then, I decided to participate in the clinical trial of a new drug (Remdesivir).* But I was assigned to the control group and kept taking the AIDS drug. ... *That was the best I could do.* I don't deny that trials are scary due to possible adverse effects. They were scary at that time. But when I searched through the materials about the new drug that the doctor had given, there were many positive appraisals and a few reports of adverse effects. ... I asked the doctor how many adverse effects I would get. The doctor said that because I was young and in my 20s, there would be few adverse effects, such as blood vessel expansion. *He persuaded me into it. I was, in fact, hoping for such encouragement.* ... When I returned to the hospital for plasma donation, I heard from researcher nurses that the Remdesivir trials led to nothing. They said that it turned out to be no cure since it had produced many adverse effects and no curative effect when applied to patients in critical conditions. ... Nurses and doctors also said that, whatever drugs I had taken during the hospitalization, it must've been my body itself and not the drugs that had made me through it all. ... Doctors and nurses said that there were no drug cures but the antibodies in the plasma of the recovered people. ... It was none of the drugs for symptomatic control but the body itself that generated antibodies that had made me recover. *Personally, I think the placebo (deception) that I had taken some drugs got me through as well.*

(Hwan)

Some people made strong complaints (about having no real cure.) *I was somewhat resigned.*

(Ree)

I got dozens of pills that were red, green, and blue. I was told to simply take them after each meal. *I didn't know what they were. In fact, I wasn't curious about them*. Now I think they were experimental pills since healthcare workers were curious about which pills had effects.

(Song)

It was suffocating to be locked in the treatment center without a cure. I took tests on a regular basis. I did my best to take the multivitamins that my family had packed for me. Eating well and drinking well was all I could do. *I was frustrated. ... I felt so helpless. ...* We were assaulted by the virus all of a sudden. The government had said we could do routine things without too many measures like border shutdown and mask mandates. I wished we had locked the border earlier, but that was not something I could have done. Many procedures should've worked better. But *I couldn't control them or get involved to make changes*. It was all *beyond my capacity*. Many people and even the government wanted something done, but it was *beyond their reach* as well.

(Jin)

As I stayed in the hospital longer than I expected, I started getting nervous. Although there wasn't any cure, they gave me some drugs as treatment. ... The AIDS pills ... we took them. But, after some time, I thought to myself and realized that *doctors were not healing me but only isolating me from the outside. That was the goal.* Those pills were not to get rid of the coronavirus, but they were experimental. *It was like they were running clinical experiments on us. So, I stopped taking the pills.*

(Cheol)

Testing Dehospitalization

While people have not taken real cures in a hospital or a community treatment center, the government's decision to free the once infected from institutional quarantine should come as a surprise. However, the dismissal from the institutions mostly takes a sluggish rather than swift course, putting those awaiting the release into another round of pendulation between two poles. On one hand, they long to take the final tests as soon as possible in which they need to get negative results two consecutive times for release; on the other, because it is not easy to get those two negative results after only the symptomatic treatments, they paradoxically feel reluctant to stand up for the final tests for fear that they would not get the desired result and get disappointed. They hope for and call forth good news at the same time as they paradoxically prep themselves up to readily suck in bad news (Min, Song, Jin, Han, Ree, Bae, and Gan). Under these pressures, some people even develop deep-seated resignation and doubt about hospital discharge (Sun and Wook).

After some time in the hospital, patients took tests every other day. If a person tested negative consecutively in two tests, the person could go home. For me, it was negative one day and positive on the next test; sometimes, it was a borderline result, somewhere between negative and positive. *Depending on the test results, my mentality swung between hope and disappointment. The hope for hospital discharge was followed by disappointment many times. It was a ruthless, repetitive process. I was disappointed as much as I expected* good results. *Even now, I don't feel like taking any test like it anymore.* … Some people hated having their nose poked with the test stick. I got used to it, and it was bearable because I had done it many times. But *the most difficult and onerous part was to wait for the test results.*

(Min)

It was two weeks after hospitalization when I started taking the daily virus tests to see if it was negative or positive. … One day, it was negative. It was positive the next day. It became negative again and then positive. *It was ridiculous.* … *I became free of symptoms after two or three weeks in the hospital.* … But *it took me and my friends 40 to 50 days to finally be discharged.*

(Song)

After two weeks, I got negative on the test. *I thought, 'I can now go home.'* But it was positive the next day. *'Again, I am stuck here one more time (after my plan to get a job was derailed due to the infection),' I thought. I was dejected.*

(Jin)

'Yes, I'm going home tomorrow,' I thought while *I was packing up* one day. Then, getting back the positive test result, *I unpacked* and got depressed.

(Han)

It was after 13 days in the hospital. I got a negative. 'I would go home if it's another negative tomorrow,' *I was uplifted.* But it was positive. *I cried.* I wanted to get out so much. I was so hammered down. … Negative turned into positive. Positive turned into negative. It was like that. I went through these switches several more times. *After a while, I didn't get emotional at those overturns.* I took them simply as they were. Nothing more. Nothing less.

(Ree)

It was like *torturing yourself toward the ever-elusive hope.*

(Bae)

It was like negative and then positive; then, another cycle of negative and positive. I went through three cycles, and ten days passed like that. *I got exhausted.* ... When I heard I would be discharged, it was truly like a dream. It was unreal. ... *I was suppressing all the hopeful thinking because I had been hit back as much as I had anticipated for a happy end.* The counter-hit had lasted for one whole day. So, I was watching TV without expecting anything when the doctor told me to pack up. It was purely jubilating.

(Gan)

The test results were pendulating from negative to positive endlessly. Then, *I doubted* that I could go home someday.

(Sun)

I was caught between negative and positive results. *I once doubted my chance to go home.*

(Wook)

Dehospitalization Without a Sense of Recovery

Once people finally acquire negative results and return to home or work, they often run into conflicting situations in which they do not feel recovered or healed in real bodily senses (Sun, Gan, Hee, Han, and Wook). The fact that they have not taken any explicit cure but symptomatic treatments reinforces these feelings. As a result, some even doubt any recovery from the infection.

> *I didn't think I was one of the cured*, because *I hadn't been treated with any cure drugs or interventions.* Nothing had gotten rid of the viruses from my body. It was okay that others called me the cured, but *it didn't feel real* to me.
>
> (Sun)

> I had that *lingering feeling of frustration* after hospital discharge. I took sleep pills for a while. The sleep problem lasted for some time. It was the most difficult backwash. ... *I kept having the same diarrhea* that I used to have while being treated in the hospital. It's special, and I knew it was somehow related to Covid-19. Although I was discharged, I had it for another week or so. *It was mysterious.* ... Occasionally, I couldn't breathe well. I didn't know why. But, in the crowded place, I wasn't breathing well. I thought it was one of the backwashes. *This breathing problem stayed with me ever since the infection.*
>
> (Gan)

Back at home, *I was utterly fatigued out.* I couldn't move around much doing the housework, as if I had lost chunks of muscle. My mom helped me a lot and took care of the kids for me. … I wasn't sure of my body. *I wasn't sure whether my body was healed.* To make it worse, there was a rumor about the once infected people turning back to the infection-positive status.

(Hee)

When I felt something wrong with my body, *I kept suspecting Covid-19 in my body.*

(Han)

There was a *remaining infection in my lung* when I was discharged. So, I took regular lung tests for two more months. … *I felt less energy in my body. It's a sense of fatigue.* It was hard to pinpoint what it was. But I seemed to have less power. If I used to pull up 80 out of 100 from my body before the infection, I couldn't do that much after the infection. It was below 80. I could still do things, but it was not with all the power that I used to fire up.

(Wook)

Being a Risk and at Risk

Doubts about the real recovery from infection are often revealed in the interviewees' perception of themselves as both being at risk and being a risk (Sook, Bae, and Hee). Risk is always two-way among them. Their self-perception is two-fold: surrounded by viruses that put them at risk and by people to whom they are a risk.

The trauma lasted long. *The fear* even after hospital discharge was enormous. Whenever I had a headache or muscle pains, I went for tests for fear of Covid-19. … I kept suspecting, '*What if I spread the virus?*' Whenever I didn't feel well, I suspected, '*Am I getting the virus again?*' … This worry made me homebound.

(Sook)

I didn't go straight home from hospital but to a hotel and stayed there for two weeks more. I voluntarily put myself in seclusion. … *I was worried about infecting my family.* … I developed claustrophobia. *I feared the places where people were jammed.* … In those places, I held tight to masks, tightened them again, and shielded my body from others. *Re-infection was dreadful.*

(Bae)

I didn't feel comfortable back at home. I kept wearing masks at home for a month, *in fear of being infected again, and infecting my family.*

(Hee)

Fragility: The Self Surrounded by Multiplex Forces

Finally, the infected experience the most fundamental aspect of liminality by encountering the fragile, vulnerable self-surrounded by and interwoven with unspecified, unaccountable, and opportunistic forces in the world. These multiple forces are daily, mundane routines – e.g., work, family reunion, church service attendance, student room sharing, socializing, xenophobia, etc. (Hee 1, Sook 1, Chang, Sun, Bae 1, Jin 1, and Seul 1); untouchable supra-individual powers – e.g., luck, unavoidable others, mysterious viruses, situations, deities, etc. (Hwan, Sung 1, Woo, Kwang, Han, Dong, Seul 2, Bae 2, Jin 2, Ree, and Hee 2); and personal, casual faults (Sung 2 and Sook 2). People mostly come to appreciate the fragility of diverse origins when they reflect on where the infectious disease has stemmed from.

Once they realize their fragility and vulnerability vis-à-vis these multiplex forces, they often end up with self-blame and personal fault-finding. Yet, they do not imply that they should and can be free from those forces and influences. Instead, they take fragility and vulnerability in front of these forces as inexorable – if not explicable easily – part of them existing in the world.

Mundane Routines

People always asked me about how I got infected. That's the first question I always got from others *as if they were imploring any unusual answer from me. But it was from part-time work.* I was a waitress at a restaurant, and one of the clients had been infected. I must've contacted him. *It just happened so.*

(Hee 1)

I had to go abroad for my daughter's wedding. My daughter and son-in-law couldn't come to Korea for the wedding, so his parents and I agreed to visit them. ... As soon as I returned home to Korea, I followed the mandate to get tested. In the evening, I got notified of the positive test result. ... *I was upset at the result. 'Why me?' I was angered.* On my return flight, I had been seated next to Italian nuns. So, I suspected they infected me. I harassed the authorities to find out whether they were accountable for my infection. On second thought, though, I might've infected them. It might've been a third person on the flight. *Who knows?*

(Sook 1)

We guessed it was at the church retreat where the infection had begun. It's only a guess because *we didn't look into where it had actually come from*. We only heard that the origin was never revealed clearly. *As usual, many fellow believers had participated in the retreat, and many of them had been infected. So, we thought it was there.* It's only conjecture, though. ... We (believers in the same church) were the first infection cases in Busan. The government eagerly conducted contact tracing to find out the first infectant, or case number 0. It didn't find it. *We settled down in accepting* that we all got infected during the worship and *didn't learn or want to learn where it started. ... We gave up and let it go.*

(Chang and Sun)

Before I returned from *study abroad*, I shared a room with two others. One of them and *I had trouble with the landlord, and we had to move out of the place and packed into that small room.* Until I got back to Korea, we lived together and relied upon one another for a while. I believe it was there where I got infected. *It was just like that.*

(Bae 1)

It didn't feel alright (that people criticized the infected people). *It didn't look fair.* I don't know how to put the feeling. *It (infection) is simply something that could've befallen anyone. ... People got infected in fleeting encounters here and there.*

(Jin 1)

I visited London from a southern city, which had been planned long ago and already paid for. It was when infection cases started being reported in the UK. So, my friends and I didn't go to many places. ... On the bus back to the southern city, people were coughing a lot all around my seat. *So, I begrudgingly put on a mask because I was the only person wearing it, if not promptly. I believe it was on the bus that I got infected. ... It was my first time wearing a mask, though.* Nobody was wearing a mask in London. There was even a recent hate crime against Asians, an assault and battery, Covid-19-related. *I, as an Asian girl, didn't feel safe about wearing a mask and running the risk of being targeted and assaulted. So, I hadn't worn it while in London.*

(Seul 1)

Supra-Individual Powers

Now I think I was *unlucky*. I also think anyone can get infected anytime *by bad luck*. I was one of those *ill-fated* people.

(Hwan)

I was usually a lucky person and had good luck in many things in all my life. But, *when I was infected, it was from bad luck.* I was sitting in a restaurant right next to a group of nine people, seven of whom turned out to be infected later on. ... But I doubted that they infected me and my friends because we hadn't talked to or eaten with them at all. ... I am not an expert. But, I suspected, and I still suspect, that I got infected actually from *the hospital, where I had to come close to those who were most likely infected to take the coronavirus test and see if the people at the restaurant had infected me. Who knows?* I reluctantly accept that I got infected at the restaurant because the authority told me so.

(Sung 1)

Corona (Covid-19) changed a lot in my life. Without it, I would be doing business there (in Dubai). The outbreak ruined my business plan. Costs and benefits didn't match. A real calamity was looming. So, I gave it up and decided to come back and live here. I was stressed out. *I thought I was doomed by bad luck.* ... I was really pissed off and upset. I got angered and infuriated. *I didn't understand why me* and why this happened to me, as those who got serious diseases often ask. ... *I blamed my bad luck. I was angry.* ... (Before I started the business) I had been an executive board member at Samsung when I retired. One morning at the year-end, I got a call saying that I didn't have to get to work the next day and ever. That's a terrible shock. It kindled anger inside me because I wasn't persuaded why I had to quit. The company wasn't and couldn't be bad business profit-wise. *So, it all came down to age. As you got older than others, you had to quit.* ... With this burden on my heart, I did my best for a new business. Then, Covid-19 broke out, and the business didn't sell much. Making matters worse, I got infected. *Can you imagine how hard it was to get hold of myself?*

(Woo)

There was a man who was believed to spread the virus to us. But *there was nothing we could do about it. It was inevitable. Nothing was wrong.* He hadn't met his father for a long time since he went abroad. So, when he came back, *he just had to meet his father (whom the man infected and who was attending the same church that I attended and subsequently infected me). Could he dare not to meet his father?*

(Kwang)

The bar owner had just returned from abroad and must've felt merry with some of her friends in the bar. We were strangers and only occasional visitors to her, but she moved around throughout the bar and *poured wine* even to us *as a courtesy. She came to our table and talked to me freely out of courtesy.* Once we learned about our infection, we blamed the bar owner. ... I had been a homebody until I went there to get some fresh air that night. I didn't drink a drop and had only a soft drink. My friends were tipsy and had fun with wine, at least. I was sober alone and drove them home. *It was a nasty blow to my face.*

(Han)

'Me being infected?' *It was senseless and clueless* ... Whatever precautions people took, it could be anybody who got infected. There was no guarantee *against these invisible viruses.* ... *Even 'the origin infectant' got infected from someone else or somewhere else.* Isn't that right? The person must've had no bad intention to spread the virus. The person must've gotten it from somewhere without even realizing it. *That person had happened* to attend my church. So, we got infected. I don't think there would've been any difference even if we had known who the origin infectant was. ... *We cannot say anything about the origin infectant who had been infected by someone else who we would never know.*

(Dong)

I didn't know where it all started. It might not be the ESL language school that I attended. The British government didn't run the coronavirus test on many of its people. *There must have been many infection cases out there, only if it had done more tests.* I assumed I was simply the first who was infected and got the test.

(Seul 2)

I was a victim to the virus. Without it, I would've had fun abroad. I was locked up for 2-3 weeks and came back. *It was unrighteous.*

(Bae 2)

I didn't want to get it. *I simply fell victim to the virus.*

(Jin 2)

I couldn't do what I had originally planned to do abroad because of the outbreak. *This made me helpless and begrudged. Situations at that time were beyond my power* and forced me to return home. Then, I ultimately got sick. *Things were coming one after another.*

(Ree)

When the infection seemed to slow down, I asked myself, '*Is that it? Is it going to end like this after I got infected and suffered alone?*' It seemed unrighteous. *Why only me?* Why not all the others? It didn't seem right. As I am a Christian, *I even blamed God a lot.* Nothing good was occurring to me. I blamed myself as well.

(Hee 2)

Casual Faults

At first, it felt unfair for others to criticize me for being infected. Who would've wanted it? At the same time, I was telling myself. *'Alas, it's my own fault. I should've been more careful. I shouldn't have gone out to be with others.'* ... But I don't know. Different people have different styles. It would've been alright if I were a homebody in personality. But *I am an outgoing type of person.* I am E in MBTI. I love meeting friends. *I couldn't help it.* ... The whole world was full of threats and fear. *I had been withholding myself until that very night when I failed* to hold it any further. I met a friend that night.

(Sung 2)

At the end of the day, it was my own fault. ... It was I who went abroad against all odds. *I had taken the risk for my personal cause to attend my daughter's wedding.*

(Sook 2)

Exposed Self, Exploded Self

According to the government policy on contact tracing, the infected are mandated to release personal information to the public. As a result, unknown others know unusual details about the infected ego, whereas the ego asymmetrically does not know or hold any control over these unknown others who can possibly do anything affecting the ego, materially and psychologically. In these power and knowledge imbalances, the exposure of the self to the outer world leads unnecessarily to the sense of the self being dissected and exploded.

The city government posted information about infection cases online. Although there was no name, people around me knew it was me based on what was posted online. *They called me to confirm. I didn't want to but had to admit I was among the infected.*

(Kwang)

Upon testing positive after returning from abroad, I was caught by great fear, especially *the fear that I would be isolated from others.* That is because, for the sake of public health, every piece of information about me was disclosed (by the government) to everyone in the city where I was living. *The information was comprehensive, so that anybody who had known me easily could guess that it was I who got infected in the city.* So, people kept calling me to confirm their guess.

(Sook)

I disclosed every possible information about my movement. ... *My home address was exposed, not exactly the street number but the street name. So, food shops refused to deliver any order* from my brother, who was not infected but stayed at my home while I was hospitalized.

(Chang)

My job, workplace, and age were disclosed. Too much of my information was released. ... I am a teacher. So, as I was working in the public sector, I cooperated with the government and disclosed a lot of information about me. ... *Student parents, my neighbors, and news reporters called me unexpectedly. ... I had to suffer from those unwanted interruptions.*

(Sung)

My information was *stored in online blogs and communities forever* under the call names like 'Osan case number X' and 'Osan case number Y.' *It never disappeared while being imprinted online like 'the Scarlet Letter.'* ... It can be temporarily disclosed for public safety. But the permanent online storing was too much.

(Han)

It was scary when the information was true. People posted details about me: *how old I was, where I lived, where I usually went, and who my friends were. It's so scary.*

(Gan)

Anonymous people reacted with negative, aggressive comments to the news reports about my infection. *I was being dominated by what these people said about me.* It was scary.

(Min)

References

Berger, P. L., & Luckmann, T. (1991 [1967]). *The social construction of reality: A treatise in the sociology of knowledge.* Penguin Books.

Simmel, G. (1908). The stranger. In K. H. Wolff (Ed. & Trans.), *The sociology of Georg Simmel* (pp. 402–408). Free Press.

Turner, V., & Turner, E. (1978). *Image and pilgrimage in Christian culture: Anthropological perspective.* Columbia University Press.

van Gennep, A. (1960 [1909]). *The rites of passage* (M. B. Vizedom & G. L. Caffee, Trans.). University of Chicago Press.

3 Plasma Donations

Koreans have donated blood plasma in reaction to the nationwide campaign run by the government health authorities, hospitals, and drug companies (Figure 3.1). The 19 interviewees have donated it once or several times after they were released from medical facilities. Most of them have visited a university-affiliated research hospital – i.e., Korea University Ansan Medical Center – to donate it from corners of the country, while a few have visited Red Cross blood donation centers in the vicinity.

When asked how they decided to donate it, donors provided a variety of causes and meanings of donation. Typically, donors bring up five different causes for initiating donation (the horizontal headings in Figure 3.2), depending on what they experience social-relationally and bio-physiologically at the time when they get infected and when they get treated in specialized facilities – i.e., ways of turning liminal. When they suffer significantly from viruses or social relations, they donate initially to build self-confidence against viruses or social-relational enmity. When they find it especially fearful and threatening to have undergone the hardship in quarantine without a real cure but only with symptomatic treatment, they report cure-making as the initial cause. When they feel thankful for emotional and material help from others in the treatment process, donors likely identify paying good for good, or goodwill repayment for goodwill help, as the initial cause. Fourth, goodwill repayment is sometimes not in return for goodwill help but social-relational enmity among some donors. These donors initiate donations to reciprocate evil with good – or to pay good for evil – primarily motivated by religious decrees and obligations. Finally, there is a fifth group of donors who embody the notion of noblesse oblige and conduct the civic duty of social responsibility in no return for goodwill help or social enmity.

In addition, donors develop various emergent meanings and causes (the vertical headings in Figure 3.2), depending on which initial causes they have embarked on donation for and what they have experienced in the experiential, context-specific unfolding of donation. Although each of the five initial causes has the potential to remain static as it is or to

DOI: 10.4324/9781003493723-4

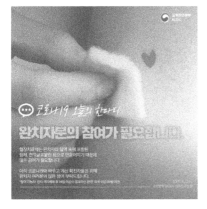 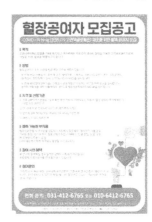

Figure 3.1 Donor Recruitment Posters by the Korea Center for Disease Control and Prevention (KCDC) (Left) and Korea University Ansan Medical Center (Right)

Note: It reads in the left poster, "Daily message from KCDC on June 3, 2020: we need many recovered people to participate in donations for developing plasma remedies for the still many infected people." The poster on the right is a more specific recruitment notice, stating the purpose of plasma donations, how to donate, who can donate, possible adverse effects, and benefits to donors.

evolve dynamically into other causes and meanings, the cause of goodwill payment for goodwill help tends to produce emergent meanings most dynamically. At the same time, however, not all cases of this cause naturally beget further meanings. It is consequential for the evolution of multiple emergent meanings whether donors are conditioned to reflect on different – pre-known and unknown – meanings of donation. Several such enabling factors are evident in the interviews: whether donors donate once or multiple times in which various causes may emerge; whether they each donate alone or with companions who may have different motivations from one another, such as coworkers, friends, family, and congregation members; and whether donors develop meaningful relationships – mostly, conversational – with the staff at the donation place who casually inform them of the dynamic changes in their bodily health as well as recent developments in the pandemic situation and the anti-pandemic medical science in the world. When none of these contextual factors are present, even the goodwill repayment cause is infertile to any emergent causes. When one or more of these factors are present, the other initial causes that are less fertile are likely to generate emergent causes.

In all, plasma donation that has been made in conscious and unconscious responses to the uncertainties and liminality that coronavirus disease-2019 (COVID-19) has caused works as another instance of liminality

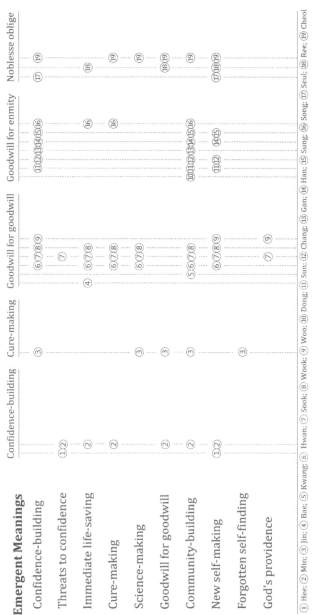

Figure 3.2 Initial Causes and Emergent Meanings of Plasma Donation, by Donors. Figure by the authors

that defies any simple, categorical signification. Donors experience divergent initial causes and appreciate various emergent meanings. Plasma donation is a dynamic process and a living fact rather than a fixed event. As a result, there are variations among donors in the kind and number of causes and meanings that they ascribe to plasma donation. Some donors refer only to a fixed set of meanings and causes that have initially driven them to donate. In contrast, others refer to an evolving set of emergent meanings and causes that they come to realize once they have participated in donation.

Confidence-Building against Viruses and Social Enmity

One of the critical experiences of liminality is worries and fears that there are no cures but only symptomatic treatment while being institutionalized in hospitals and community care centers (i.e., the "treatment with no cure" code in Chapter 2). Upon discharge from these facilities, therefore, people naturally wonder if they have recovered in the real sense (i.e., the "dehospitalization without a sense of recovery" code). In addition, people have experienced the fragility of the self, surrounded by multiple unavoidable forces in the world (i.e., the "fragility amid multiplex forces" code). To those, plasma donation comes first as a test to tell if one has recovered from the infection and carries enough antibodies. Thus, plasma donation is part of confidence-building in a biological sense. To this very extent, however, it ironically means to run the risk of finding oneself possibly not endowed with sufficient antibodies. Some donors even learn that plasma drawing is so much a risky adventure that strains the still-recovering body. Hee provides a typical story. Although Hee donates to build her confidence in health, she comes to realize that plasma donation is a threat as well as a boon for confidence-building. To Hee, both plasma donation and writing have ambivalent effects on her effort to regain self-confidence.

> *I wasn't sure of my body. I wasn't sure whether my body was healed.* To make it worse, there was a rumor about the once infected people turning back to their infection-positive status. I had to look after my kids and continue daily business with others. I was worried about how I could ever go on with this body. *I needed confidence in myself. I needed to confirm that my body was completely healed. So, I went for plasma donation,* I think. ... After *I took the pretest to see if I could donate plasma,* it took about 1-2 months until I finally donated it. In the meantime, I was only hoping to donate as soon as possible. I wanted to confirm that I wasn't going to infect others. *It was an awfully long wait.* My kids were not going to school but stayed home with me all day. It was difficult. ... *When I finally learned that my blood had enough antibodies*

and my body was no longer at risk, I was delighted. ... Because I knew I was not suitable for (ordinary) blood donation because of iron deficiency, *I took iron supplements daily and drank fluid extracts of a black goat to make this plasma donation happen.* I was a children's book storyteller. Unless *I proved myself to others with plasma donation,* I wouldn't be able to stand before them as a storyteller. ... *Plasma donation helped me a lot.* I could take myself not as the host of viruses but as a normal person. *I got comforted quite a bit by the fact that I had antibodies.* ...

I knew my plasma would be used for research but didn't know how exactly. The researchers must've used it right. *I didn't really care.* ... Months after the first donation, I heard that I was still carrying antibodies. But *I didn't feel I was healthy enough to make another donation. Blood drawing seemed to strain my body.* ... *I wasn't feeling completely recovered from the disease.* You know we need some time to recover fully from childbirth. I was feeling just that way, psychologically and physically. I had lost muscles during the hospitalization, and I was getting tired easily. ... *It was like how I felt about writing.* When I was hospitalized, I wrote down what I had felt since my infection. Recently, I put them together into a book only for myself. I did so because I thought I had overcome all the difficult feelings by listening to them and writing them down. *I had learned in the hospital that I could overcome my suffering not by neglecting it but by acknowledging it and writing about it.* That's how I kept writing about my experiences and shared them on the blog with other infected people hospitalized at that time. *But when I was working on the book publication (for only two copies), those hard feelings and trauma came back alive.* They didn't go away completely. *My heart was thumping inside.*

(Hee)

Confidence-building is also directed to social relations, to the extent that other key experiences of liminality are estrangement – ego-initiated and alter-initiated – and fragility vis-à-vis multiple forces involving social relations in mundane routines. Plasma donation is an effective way for those who intend to overcome social enmity toward them since it attests that the infected are not only back to normal but stand as benevolent donors for others. However, donors realize that this potential gain is not without a cost. Donors who have once suffered from others' criticism must put themselves together and expose themselves to others' evaluation one more time. In this sense, plasma donation becomes both an opportunity for and a threat to confidence-building in a social-relational sense.

While in hospital, I got cuts on my heart from the online posts about me. I didn't get infected because I did something wrong. But *people kept criticizing me, putting me in big fear (of others I shouldn't have dreaded). So, I kept hiding away; I was heartbroken and depressed. …* I didn't want it that way. I didn't want the criticism to go on and hurt me. *I wanted to heal myself. Then, I saw the news about plasma donation. …* After the donation, I might've wanted to boast about it. *It testified that I didn't yield to the fear of others, their negative looks, and criticism of me, and instead, I tackled the problem (infection and others' reaction) in a good way. I might've wanted to tell them I did it my way.* 'How could I think about it (plasma donation as well as diary-keeping) while I was still in the hospital' I asked myself. I didn't get a definite answer. *I might've wanted others to see that I solved the problem in my (unforeseen but good) way. … I told people who knew I had been infected that I got antibodies. …*

It wouldn't be easy for all to decide to donate plasma because it would then remind donors of all the prejudiced criticisms and difficulties. *Who could easily stand out for donation at the risk of being blamed again? …* But *I had a strong desire to see that I was okay, and I made the donation. …* Most people might've wanted to hide away one more time. … *As the mother of two kids, I had the guts. …* At the same time, I haven't decided whether I will publish it (a collection of writings on her experiences during hospitalization) to the public since I am scared that people who haven't known about my infection and all would know it all. Then, I would have to *confront those difficult emotions in front of others one more time.*

(Hee)

I don't think we can criticize those who recovered and decided not to donate. I think donation is good. But these people can have different situations. When they were infected, they must've undergone difficult situations and emotions, like negative reactions from around. … *These things might've blocked them from donating. (Plasma donation might remind them of these difficulties.) … It might remind them of the hurts and trauma once more.*

(Jin)

When I went to the street donation center – which Red Cross ran, the staff looked at me in surprise. It seemed that she hadn't expected any donors. She said that most recovered people were unwilling to donate because any volunteers would be background-checked in the national health information system, and *it would expose once more when and how they had been infected, treated, and released from quarantine. Not many people would go through it once again.* Thanks to the background check, I re-learned my exact dates of hospitalization and dehospitalization. … Once released from quarantine facilities, people wanted to take themselves as being back to normal. That's very plausible. I did so, too. But, *when you stepped into the plasma donation place, you were like proclaiming yourself to others as someone who had been infected and recovered but not really normal. ... This could be a difficult decision* for some people, although I didn't hesitate to step up.

(Bae)

Interestingly, the affirmation that plasma donation has conflicting and contradictory potentials for confidence-building has led some donors (e.g., Hee) to realize an emergent cause in plasma donation that donors have not foreseen beforehand. Once living through the dual meanings of dona-tion, Hee is awakened to a new self – i.e., new self-making – who becomes no longer troubled by contradictions and ambivalences that were unac-ceptable in the past. In the following quote, Hee reveals the unexpected personal growth in accepting the hard-to-take contradiction between what she intends to deliver to others and what others actually receive from her and the contradiction between how she hopes to lead her life and how she is actually allowed to. As much as she embraces two conflicting mean-ings of plasma donation, she accepts two contradictory attitudes in her relationships with others and even the duality of human nature in her and others. She admits that these are explicit moments of personal growth.

Going through infection and plasma donation, I came to understand others in a broader lens. ... I had been overly concerned with how others would think of me and how I would be viewed in their eyes. But, after the event, *I realized that I could live my life as I liked it. It was I that was the most important. Whatever I did, I realized, people took it as they liked to. I came to accept that I could live my life in a selfish way. ... It's an irony. I realized no event had simply one meaning. ... I am soft-voiced and shy. But I'm also bold and gutsy. ...* I learned that there were not many people who were so commonsensical and righteous as I had believed. So, I let go of many of my good old expectations about other people. *I shouldn't have looked up to others so much as I had been doing, even though I cared about these people. ...* Don't get me wrong. I liked to meet people. I still do. I hang out with people and share things quite of-ten. After the event, I mean, I only met people who liked me and didn't stress me out. In the past, I had worked so hard to be nice to all people. I had wanted to be taken as a good person by all. But I realized it didn't have to be that way. ... At the moment, there are people I don't under-stand. But, in the course of time, I believe I can understand them and may want to meet them, not only the believers at my church (whom I have not always felt comfortable being with) but those who hurt my feelings deliberately or not when I was suffering from Covid-19. *The bottom line is nobody is perfect, like my apartment neighbors who criticized me for being infected and harmful to them but welcomed my story because it got their apartments nationwide attention and pushed up the market recognition.* We are all the same. I came to know that. At times, I simply wasn't able to accept those people because I wasn't in the mindset. When I find peace in my heart again, I will be able to smile and meet those people. *I accept it all.*

(Hee)

Min's story shows a more dynamic evolution of emergent meanings than Hee. Like Hee, Min has initially conceived of plasma donation to build self-confidence in front of other people and the still circulating viruses. Once she has started it, she has fully appreciated the contradictory meanings involved in plasma donation.

When *I first stumbled upon the internet ad about plasma donation,* I was having a difficult time running daily routines. It wasn't easy to go out and meet friends. I mostly stayed in my room. When I saw the ad, *I thought donation could be a way to break down this trauma.* So, I decided to go for it. Then, I heard I had to go through the Covid-19 test to donate, and *I got scared at the thought of the test. A week passed in hesitation.* ... I called the hospital to ask if I could donate without the test. The hospital made an exception for me, and I immediately arranged for a donation. I took a pretest to check my bodily condition and antibodies. *I was so anxious about the pretest result that I couldn't sleep well for two days until I heard the result.* Two weeks after I got the pretest result, I donated my plasma. ...

Before the donation, I was suffering a lot psychologically. I even thought that I wouldn't be able to live any longer with those people in this country who knew me. *Not until I met the hospital staff for donation had I met any strangers ever since my release from quarantine several months ago.* ... I was finally able to talk to strangers (i.e., the hospital staff), and it helped me. They took me, the once infected, as nobody special. It was my first time being treated as a plain individual. They applauded my donation, and *it comforted me psychologically, while my donation must've benefited them. It helped me break down my trauma (from the Covid-19 infection) about 80%, if not completely.* After the first donation, *I was relieved a lot and could try something else. I overcame the hardship thanks to my donation.* ... *I Instagrammed that I overcame the trauma.* I hadn't talked about the trauma even to my friends before. Instagramming was the first time letting them know about it and plasma donation. *I wrote about how I overcame it with the donation.* Then, Instagramming helped me to overcome it further. ... *If I hadn't donated it then, I wouldn't have overcome the trauma easily.* I might've needed more time. ... *After donating, I felt I was finally back among people.*

(Min)

Once Min has participated in plasma donation, she comes to encounter other diverse emergent causes in donations, such as new self-making (accepting blood donation that her old self never embraced), community-building (with her infected mom who joins her in participating in the donation drive), cure-making, immediate life-saving, and goodwill repayment for goodwill help. She has donated two times and wants to continue it.

After the first donation, Korea University (authors' note: KU, hereafter) Hospital told me that I had a high level of *antibodies* compared to other donors. *I felt smug.* I felt like I got paid back for what I had suffered from infection. *Then, one day, another university hospital contacted me* through KU Hospital to ask if I could donate plasma for a critically ill Covid-19 patient there. *So, I did it again. … I had never done even the ordinary blood donation before* because my whole family has low blood pressure. That is why *my mom had initially discouraged me* from plasma donation. But I did it because the pretest results gave me a green light. After I did it once, I felt like I could do it again. I wanted to do it whenever I was asked to. *I got over the fear of blood donation. … It's interesting. After my donation, my mom also donated her plasma.* After she saw that donation involved some benefits like a pretest on bodily condition and antibody measurement, she followed me. But she still rebuked me for my second donation. …

I didn't know plasma was not blood-colored but yellow. It was so unfamiliar that I wanted to touch and feel it. The staff allowed me to take photos of it, which I kept for memory. *I felt so proud of myself* when the staff took it to freeze and store it. … When I heard my plasma would be directly injected into a patient in the ICU, I felt even more proud. My first donation was for me to check my body and for the hospital to develop pharmaceutical cures supported by the government. *As for the second donation, the hospital unexpectedly called me first for an emergency transfusion to the ICU patient. I heard it was the last hope the patient had. So, I agreed. …*

I had hated being confined in quarantine, and it had been such a long process. So, I believe *I wanted nobody to go through such a time as I did. Part of me was telling it once I began donating. I seemed to expect cure drugs to be developed,* as well. … *I also wanted to pay back* for the help and support that I had received during my infection treatment in the hospital.

(Min)

Cure-Making

The experience of treatment with no cure prompts people to develop anxiety over the intractable pandemic situation, which drives them to donate their plasma to treat immediate patients in critical conditions and, ultimately, to develop reliable real cures. The following excerpt from Jin is exemplary.

I had been so focused on myself due to psychological sufferings that I was having from relations like family. Over the course of time, I realized the hard work and help of healthcare workers at the treatment center. I was grateful to them. *When I first heard about the development plan for plasma treatment, I wanted to be of help and part of it* as soon as possible. When I asked a nurse about it, she said I could donate it several times at a proper interval. So, I made donation reservations myself and made *donations five times. … I was so desperate. I hoped to see a real cure made* from the plasma that I donated. I have been watching the news about it since I started donating. I thought it would be really great if my blood could be used for that cause. That was what made me keep donating continuously. … It didn't feel good to draw blood out and put it back into my body. But my hope that this (the pandemic) should end as soon as possible was greater than the strange feeling. I hoped my small involvement in this to be of help. … When I tested positive, I was living with my mom, an older sister, her husband, and their kids. So, all of them had to take the tests because of me. … I felt really, really sorry for the family. I hoped nobody ever needed to go through it like I did. But I knew the infection would spread to other healthy people, and they would suffer, sometimes unnecessarily, like I did. I knew what people had to suffer. *I didn't want that happening to anybody. I only hoped somebody to make a cure (out of the plasma.) That was my only wish.* …

I had mixed feelings about the fact that we were all facing a new era where we were engulfed by the ever-spreading viruses but couldn't do anything about them at our own will. Then, doctors were trying to develop a real cure by using the plasma that people donated. *I was surprised that I was facing such a new era, and we were all facing a turning point.* It was not only me. It was a difficult time for all, but we had to live through it. *I had to do something.* That was it, when I am thinking about it now. … *I read news about the efficacy of plasma being debated.* I just hope for more good news about it. … People were taking vaccines but doubted their effects. That made me really sad. Then, I searched for news about plasma treatment. *I was ready to donate my plasma as many times as necessary.* … It was the first time seeing *this yellow blood* from my body. I had never seen it before. So, I took a picture of it. … In doing all this, *I hoped my original intention was carried in my blood.*

(Jin)

Once donors start donating to make cures, they often discover and develop other meanings in donation as they repeat donations, such as community-building among the once-infected donors, community-building with medical professionals, science-making, for-gotten self-finding, and new self-making. Jin's following story shows that a set of emergent causes and meanings are evolving from the ini-tial cause for donation, which seems to be driven by her "desperate" pursuit of cures via repeated donations. Her desperation results, in turn, from her realization that she and her close family have suffered a lot, and anybody will do so anytime in the absence of real cures.

It was the last donation. The university hospital (KU Ansan Center) staff asked me if *they could video-record me for broadcasting to recruit more donors*, probably because I had been donating 3 or 4 times al-ready and was with a close friend who had donated plasma with me three times. *The staff wanted to video-record both of us. So, we did it.* …

Whenever I visited there, *nurses always gave me sweet pies and choco-late bars* after donation to fill up the 'sugar level' in my body. I enjoyed them a lot. *They were the same nurses throughout my repeated visits for donations. Every time, they welcomed me with friendly greetings. That was how I kept donating.* …

When I had been donating plasma at Korea University Ansan Hos-pital several times, Seoul National University Medical Center where I had been treated for Covid-19 contacted me and asked if *I wanted to join its research project to see if I was still carrying antibodies. I conceded* because *I wanted to learn about the science* underlying donations. I had not been told about exactly how long antibodies could remain in my body *while I was donating plasma at KU*. I had simply assumed that I had them enough. …

I used to donate blood when I was in my 20s, about once every two years. Then, ever since I started paid work, I stopped it. When I went to KU Medical Center for plasma donation, *it was about ten years after the last blood donation. So, I was a little uneasy about the needle poking into the skin*. I didn't know anything about plasma donation. Surpris-ingly, *I actually felt at home* the next day after the first donation. I was concerned about whether I could continue donating. … But it was okay from the second donation onward. *I got used to it like the old days when I had made regular blood donations.* …

Due to plasma donation, I learned that I had antibodies. Antibodies in my body were not foolproof protection against the disease. Instead, *it provided a moment for many changes in my life*. I looked back on how I had lived health-wise. I became closer to my family and felt thank-ful for their loving me. The coronavirus infection wasn't simply a bad and difficult time in my life. … Every six months, the health authority called me and checked on my mental health to see if I was suffering from any psychological troubles. … *Thanks to plasma donation*, I didn't suffer much. Instead, *I became optimistic*. That was why I donated it a few more times, I think. … At my current workplace, I always see the ad about plasma donation in the elevators. I talk to myself, 'I've been there, and I have antibodies.' When I meet somebody who has unnecessarily negative views about the current disease situation, *I stand up and correct the person with objective facts about the disease. I let them know what they should know without prejudice. ... Plasma donation was something that I could do to help others. It was something that kept me continuing to find ways to get out of the difficulties. ... I was very egocentric.* I was so even among the family. I cared about what I had to do and didn't look into others' business. *But I became concerned with what others did in my family since then. ... Plasma donation made me look around.*

(Jin)

Goodwill Repayment for Goodwill Help ("Paying Good for Good")

The most frequent cause for donation is donors' willingness to pay back for the kindness and support that they have received from the staff in hospitals or community care centers. It is mostly an expression of gratitude and repayment (Jin and Bae). This motivation to reciprocate goodwill helps with goodwill donations most often ramifies into other causes during donation. Donors refer to various new causes and meanings emerging from this initial cause. However, the initial cause does not necessarily evolve into emergent meanings in some cases. One possible reason is the lack of communication between donors and the staff in blood donation centers on the street regarding donors' health conditions and daily concerns (Bae and Kwang), compared to the university medical centers that are equipped with additional technologies and human resources that facilitate donor–staff interactions (Sook and Hwan). When donors' interaction with the staff at facilities does not lead donors to various information and social relations that the donated plasma implies, donors tend to limit what donations mean to the initial causes. This stagnation happens even to those who donate repeatedly. Although repeated donations are conducive to generating new, emergent meanings and causes among donors compared to one-time donations, all repeated donations do not result in evolving meanings when donors have limited interaction with the staff at the donation place (Bae and Kwang).

Kwang's case insinuates another context in which the initial cause for donation, or the good-for-good repayment motivation, has not developed into emergent causes. Kwang donates it as he participates in the collective donation drive among fellow Christians. In other words, he donates as one of the Christians in his church community rather than one lone, unaffiliated person. For these donors, community-building among fellow Christians is another initial cause parallel to the good-for-good repayment cause. Depending on how this collective donation drive unfolds and how interactions among fellow believers fan out, therefore, Kwang is conditioned to ascribe more or fewer emergent meanings to donation. As it turns out, the collective donation drive has not proceeded as it was initially planned; donors each have donated individually at street blood donation centers but not at a university medical center; there have not been enough interactions among fellow Christian donors, and he does not find any evolving meanings in donation other than the initial cause of goodwill repayment.

> When young, we used to donate blood for movie tickets and believed our donated blood would be of help to somebody if we didn't know exactly how it helped others. *This time, when I donated plasma, I think I was simply thankful for being released healthy* from the hospital while others were dying of the disease.
>
> (Jin)

> I had this in mind. *(When I was in Turkey, I saw local people mistreating Asians like me as viruses.) When I needed to fly back home, it was not easy to get a flight, and the Korean consulate helped me a lot. When I was back, the government did all the care I needed for free.* The staff did their best. So, I had this willingness to give something helpful back to them. *I had been waiting for the slightest possibility that I could give back what I had received.* A friend (Hwan) said he donated plasma right after he got released from the hospital. But I couldn't because there were no facilities to take in donors in my city, Busan. It had to be either in Ansan (Korea University Medical Center) or Daegu (three university hospitals) at the time, which was too far. I waited several months until donation centers opened in Busan. As soon as I heard they opened, I donated. *There was only one person who donated before I did. I wanted to give back what I had received.* ... I knew that two or three donors' plasma could be used for treating one patient. *So, at the minimum, I wanted to donate two or three times. I had been saved, and I counted it as one life saved. I wanted to save one other life in return. In Turkey, I wouldn't have received any care. But, back in Korea, I thought I received very attentive care.* Doctors were around 24 hours. I had three meals a day in the hospital. *I was so thankful* for that. I had a lot of help and kindness. What I could do in return was to donate. At that moment, it was the only thing I could do. Yes, the donations made me feel that *I finally repaid my gratitude.* I am a pay-back-whatever-I-receive type of person. ...
>
> I donated at *a street blood donation center* but not a hospital. *So, I couldn't know anything about antibodies in my body, although I was so curious.* I heard from Hwan that the university hospital where he donated let him know much about his bodily condition. At the donation center in my city, they didn't do the pretest but simply took donations from volunteers who were discharged from the hospital

three months ago or more. I asked the center, but it said it didn't know anything about antibodies or others. ... I donated twice so far and would've done it more times if the center had continued taking donations.

(Bae)

Someone posted a donation suggestion on the Kakao group chat room shared by fellow believers of my church who had been infected. As soon as I read the suggestion, I thought it a good opportunity. After all, the government had paid thousands of millions of wons (tens of thousands of US dollars) for each of us. *Medical professionals, the government, Korean society, and other church members had helped us with all their hearts and hands. 'Why not help them back? Isn't there any way to pay back?' I had been thinking.* Once the suggestion was posted, many others immediately conceded. *I realized that many others had the same intention to pay back. This is how I decided to join the donation drive.* ... I had donated whole blood over 20 times, and it was my first time for plasma donation. *Compared to whole blood donation, plasma donation took about one hour, which was too long and bothersome. It was so disturbing that I was telling myself that I wouldn't donate plasma anymore.* I had thought it would take 5 minutes like the usual whole blood donation, but it took me one hour. It was so unfamiliar that I was obsessed with inconvenience and didn't think about what it meant to me otherwise. ...

(The donation process didn't go as it had been planned initially.) I had volunteered for the collective donations in June but donated individually in October. *Originally, fellow believers and I had planned to donate collectively according to a possible agreement between a high-profile research hospital and our church. But things got twisted* –no hospitals in Busan accepted donors then. In October, *we decided to donate individually at street blood donation centers* and shared the news in the group chat room. So, my first donation was seven and a half months after I got released from quarantine, and I thought another donation wouldn't be meaningful because *I wasn't sure whether I would have enough antibodies for the second round.* In fact, *the staff at the donation center suggested that antibodies would decrease in time and a second donation wouldn't be necessary.* ... *I thought one donation was enough to show symbolically that I did something.* And I believed there would be other donors who recovered more recently. I wished that my first donation had been made as planned. I could've made another donation, then. ... As the donation was made not collectively but individually at a street blood donation center, *I wasn't informed of exactly what my plasma was going to be used for.*

(Kwang)

Other than these, most cases of donation as goodwill repayment for goodwill help evolve into new, emergent causes and meanings among donors. Even Kwang, who has donated in a relatively unfavorable circumstance, admits that the donation he has made out of the repayment cause functions as an opportunity for him to experience an unpredicted, emergent meaning of donation, that is, confidence-building in front of others who seem unfriendly to him. Other cases (Hwan, Sook, Wook, and Woo) show more explicitly that the repayment cause dynamically concretizes into a variety of new meanings of plasma donation, such as confidence-building, new self-making (awakening to new self), cure-making, immediate life-saving, future science-making, community-building with medical professionals as well as fellow donors, and God's providence-realizing.

I was so frustrated by others' unapproving and aggressive prejudices toward me as one of the early infected. *I was able to get over the frustration a little, thanks to the plasma donation I made with fellow believers in the church.* ... When my story was broadcast, people replied to me and showed thankfulness for my donation and sympathy for my suffering. I was glad to see those people who sympathized with me and didn't treat me as a criminal.

(Kwang)

The medical bill for my infection treatment was over twenty million wons (about 20,000 US dollars). But I paid only nine thousand wons (about 9 dollars) out of my pocket, and the rest was paid by *tax money*. And I wasn't busy and was taking college courses at home online. *I thought it legit and dutiful to take time off my day and donate.* ... If I had been in the governmental office to design the national donation protocol, I would've made donation *mandatory* for all people who had recovered with the government's financial support. ... I volunteered for donations continuously, three times in total. First in July, and second, and third in August. *I called the hospital and volunteered for the first two donations.* I heard that they were for medical experiments to develop pharmaceutical cures. For the third donation, though, the hospital called me first and asked for my help to treat an infected old lady in her 80s in the ICU with my plasma. *The hospital texted me in the morning that the old lady was in critical condition. As soon as I got the text, I called back and ran to the hospital for a donation.* ...

When I returned to the hospital for the first plasma donation, I heard from research nurses that the Remdesivir trials (that I had participated in during hospitalization) had led to nothing. They said that it turned out to be no cure since it had produced many adverse effects and no curative effect when applied to patients in critical conditions. ... *Nurses and doctors also said that, no matter what drugs I had taken during the hospitalization, it must've been my body itself* and not any drugs that had made me through it all. ... Doctors and nurses said that there were no drug cures but the antibodies in the plasma of the recovered people. ... *It was none of the drugs for symptomatic control but the body itself that generated antibodies that had made me recover. ... I was relieved very much* when I learned that my antibody level indicated 300 on the test for my first donation. They said the cut point to determine whether there were enough antibodies was 20. The research nurse said she was surprised at my number, the second highest (to 1,000 from another person) among the cases she had known so far. She joked that I didn't even need a mask thanks to the exceptionally high level of antibody formation. *I was sort of a supercarrier of antibodies.* I had probably hoped for it. ... *If I hadn't donated, I would've never known* about antibodies in me and would've stayed anxious about being infected again. ... The regulations said we could donate every two weeks, and *I was considering frequent donations because I was pretty uplifted by my antibody level.* Then, the research nurse one day called me for my help, referring to the number. She said that it was either me or another lady (Sook) who recorded an even higher number whom she could turn to for emergency plasma transfusion. ...

I felt self-satisfied with the first two donations because I felt like I did something for this country. *I felt even more self-satisfied* with the third donation because it was about saving one real life directly. ... *Thanks to the donations, I was able to do the 'Covid coming out.'* Just like it was not easy for gays and lesbians to disclose their identities in this country, it took a lot of courage for me to disclose to others that I had been infected. My parents had called me in the hospital to deter me from informing my friends of my infection in fear of prejudiced maltreatment from others. *While I was talking about my plasma donation in SNS, I was finally disclosing my infection story in front of others. ... SNS posting has become an essential part of me now.*

(Hwan)

I couldn't but blame myself for infection. But the government provided all the treatment and care for me. I was so thankful. That's why I went for plasma donation. ... I felt obliged to donate it and wanted to help make vaccines (cures) soon and terminate the pandemic. ... *I felt peaceful in my heart when I finally donated it.* It was *as if I had paid back my debt.* ... When I was making the usual whole blood donation, it was out of a simple logic that somebody has to stock up blood for whoever falls in danger. It was without much reflection. I did it sometimes out of the general religious faith in neighborly love. *But this time, I donated plasma clearly out of gratitude to this country and its medical professionals.* I felt so proud of 'K Medicine' (authors' note: what Koreans called the allegedly successful government responses to Covid-19 approvingly). *'This is a great nation,' I thought. We Koreans were doing our best to fix things instead of criticizing and complaining.* ...

Speaking of the number that measured the level of *antibodies in me*, I was told it was around 1,200, whereas it was 300 or 400 among other healthy donors. So, the staff said that they decided to call me for help instead of asking three or four other donors. So, *I went there four times* until the hospital decided to abort the plasma project. Whenever I visited, they called me *the super-carrier* of antibodies. ... When I first learned about the exceptionally large number of antibodies in me, *I felt exhilarated, thankful, and more motivated to donate.* 'Wow, I am of great help to them. *Isn't this great for me, who once was caught in despair and fear?'* I thought. I was so thankful for myself being able to help. I hadn't been donating blood since the last time I did it when I was young. As I got older, I had been under a lot of stress at the daycare center I owned and *had been thinking I wasn't very healthy.* ... It usually took one hour to complete one plasma donation. But it took me only 20-25 minutes. *It was surprising, the staff said. It was delightful, I thought.* ...

It (plasma) was yellowish but not red. It was eye-opening. *I marveled at doctors and medicine. It was fabulous* to see them take blood out and put it back in my body. *I admired them. 'Wow, we are living with such advanced medicine,' I thought.*

And I thought, 'Am I not a healthy person, in fact, seeing that I have exceptionally rich antibodies and can donate them a lot quicker than others, in less than 30 minutes?' *I used to think I was weak in health and might develop cancer someday.* I had been living that way for a long time. *I had been in fear. But, thanks to the donations, I realized and was awakened that I was a very healthy person. This awakening gave me a totally new sense of vigor.* Being delighted, I talked to a few close friends about it and took *pride in myself.*

I was part of the effort making future medicine and science. ... As much as I gained self-confidence, I could enhance my *patriotism and love* for this country. ... I was glad that I could do something for those who were infected. *I wanted somebody, like the doctor at the donation hospital, to speed up the research with my plasma and finish this pandemic for good.* My daughters are both abroad. I used to visit them at least once a year. I hoped to bring those visits back to my routine as soon as possible. I had exceptionally rich antibodies. That must've been a great help to the research. It seems an exaggeration, but *I thought that I was helping the whole of humanity with my plasma.* ...

My two daughters living abroad got excited about my rich antibodies and the unexpectedly good health of their mom. They might've had pity on me, who lived alone and doubted my health status. Then, *after they learned about my good health through the donation episode (I had one day bragged about it in an uplifted voice), they seemed to feel relieved about their lone mom. That was great. … My mom and dad had died of cancer. So, I had been suspecting I'd get cancer for many years.* It's a shame, but I had bought several extra insurance policies in anticipation of cancer. It's only recently that I started refunding these policies, thanks to my renewed faith in God. *I believed God wouldn't let me suffer cancer and ill health.* It was a critical moment. *Then, I had these surprising experiences of plasma donation, like rich antibodies and healthy bodily conditions for donation.* No matter what doctors said about infection and plasma donation, I took it from my religious perspective, as *God meant it for me. My life became full of joy, gratitude, confidence, and vigor. …*

As I was talking about Covid with doctors and nurses at the donation hospital, I could eliminate some of the fear I had about Covid. … The hospital offered *an honorarium* for my donation. I felt very indebted and wouldn't receive it. The staff was so insistent. So, I took it and bought with the money bakery and drinks for my next donation visit. I shared the *food with the staff.* It was so rewarding that they acknowledged my gift, and I acknowledged their hard work that way. *It was joyful and fun.*

(Sook)

In the hospital, I was telling myself that *I wanted to be of help to doctors and nurses because they put every possible effort into helping me. It was moving as well as reassuring* to hear the hospital staff telling me not to feel sorry or indebted to them because *it's their calling to look after me.* In addition, my medical bill of 4 to 5 million wons (about four thousand US dollars) was paid by the government. *I wasn't sure of what exactly I could do for them, though.* Then, I saw the news about plasma donation to develop cures.

To be honest, though, it took me some time to decide to go for it after I first saw the ad. It wasn't because I was unwilling to help or because I didn't want to spare time for it, but because it was burdensome to return to the hospital. I was reluctant to go back there. At that time, the hospital meant the 15 days that I had had to spend in quarantine, locked up inside the window. That's why. Then, I learned that not many people were donating. There was only one hospital in Seoul for taking donors, the KU Ansan Hospital, and medical professionals were having a difficult time due to few donors. I thought I would regret it if I neglected it. …

The first donation was for research purposes. In May, I donated the second time upon the hospital's request, which was for an emergency transfusion to an 80-some-old patient in critical condition. *After the first donation, I felt like I had committed my body to the whole wide world, and I felt fulfilled.* The second donation was urgent. I didn't think much about it beforehand because the staff called in a hurry looking for type B blood plasma. Afterward, the second donation, in fact, *gave me a novel sentiment.* If the first one gave me a fulfilling sense in a broad and vague manner, the second donation gave me a real feel of it. *It was fulfilling and real to me.* I had seen people dying of Covid-19 in the same room when I was in the hospital. My second donation was for one such person. It was to save someone's life. *That was so great, something more than simply gratifying. It was telling me that I was somebody who could save life.*

It's not only that. *I experienced other unique moments while I was donating.* ... I met two other donors at the donation hospital. It was delightful to see them there, and I felt sympathetic to them. *Donors readily sympathized with one another. 'Hey, you suffered as I did, and yet you look great in donating as I do,' I thought.* ... Each donation took an hour, and *the staff kept talking to me about many different things.* They were always encouraging me by saying that I was giving great help. They said they were grateful and sorry for having asked for help. In fact, it was I who had been thankful to the professionals. *I thought my donation was dutiful, but they saw it as courteous.* ... The interactions with the hospital staff during donations *nurtured me with a sound knowledge of Covid-19.* So, I was able to tell apart false and authentic information. I learned how I could react to the pandemic situation with a proper attitude. I willingly shared these with others because I thought I should set an example for people. ...

It also felt great to experience the frontline medical technology that hadn't been marketized yet in the donation hospital and to meet and talk with the famous professor who was featured on TV as a leading expert about Covid-19. I received his autograph, and he said *I was making a great contribution to the fight against Covid-19.* The professor even told me that my plasma looked perfect for medical research since it was clear yellow. *It made me wish for an effective cure. These experiences made me realize that I was being helpful to our society.* Compared to conventional blood donation, plasma donation seemed to be on *a bigger scale* because it was *in the university hospital.* It took longer. *I was taking it as something deeper* than blood donation. *It was different from common blood donation.* ...

Donations made me feel fulfilled. And that feeling seemed to be evolving into other things. This succession seemed all positive to me. Although I had suffered from Covid-19, if I hadn't suffered and hadn't donated plasma, that sense of fulfillment wouldn't have been that much. I would've simply felt I recovered. *Thanks* to donations, I didn't end up simply recovering, but I expanded my spectrum of life. Plasma donation was one of the big events in my life. My outlook on the world became wider. I used to have prejudices about pockets of Korean society and medical professionals about which I hadn't had direct experiences. I then realized that I should get rid of them. ...

Once others learned about my donations, they spoke highly of me. *I used to hide away as if I had had a complex. But, after the donations, I found myself confident in speaking out about what I had been through.* ... I hadn't thought deeply about me influencing others before. I had simply hoped for good consequences for those who happened to be around me vaguely. After the donations, though, *I ended up believing that I could produce good things for others and that good things could ripple across.* ... *The process all the way to the donations was pivotal in my life.*

(Wook)

I had been hospitalized for 15 days and realized that *the Korean healthcare system was quite well-established. Hospital workers were nice and devoted*, and the government spent the national health budget for me. To make up for the national revenue that I had used up, I donated twice. *I took pride, self-satisfaction, and gratitude from it* if others didn't recognize it. ...

I did it out of goodwill. Without goodwill, it would've been impossible. To donate, donors had to reveal themselves. But most people didn't like to expose them *because it's shameful and hurts self-respect.* That's why I called the hospital for donations *secretly* without telling anyone. After the donations, I told only close friends about it. ...

The first one was voluntary, while the hospital asked for the second. It said that my antibodies were several times stronger than others'. ... *I was glad to hear about strong antibodies* and thought it was thanks to the regular exercise that I kept doing. *My kids were happy to find out about my donations and relieved* about my health because they had been shocked at my infection and deeply worried about me. ... I thought it was more valuable than standard blood donation that I was doing a couple times a year. Although the nurse didn't explain it in detail, I *overheard* that my second donation was for transfusion to a critically ill patient. She said my blood was strong enough for it. I was happy to hear it. ...

After the two donations, I went back to Dubai (where I had been working to set up my own business) and, after one month, closed my shop terminally. *After I got back, I called the hospital because I wanted to make another plasma donation.* But, it stopped accepting donations and gave me an alternative place where I could donate instead. I didn't feel like calling there and didn't donate anymore. *Instead, I made a whole blood donation* at a public health office. 'It's better than simply idling away my days,' I thought because I remained unemployed and had much free time after my early retirement from lifelong employment at Samsung. ...

One positive affirmation led to another positive affirmation. They then dispersed the negative mindsets and depression that I was going through, like other middle-aged Korean men in their 50s who were forced to retire early and feared being out of a job with nothing to do daily. *I needed to motivate myself, and there was plasma donation. It helped me focus and reclaim my worth. It was satisfying and motivating.* ... Plasma donation was a kind of self-motivation. *It was the moment to motivate myself out of bad luck toward a different future.* I felt satisfied with my life because plasma donation was something good and kept generating a positive mentality. ... In the second round of my life after early retirement, I first had bad experiences. Then, *plasma donation got me out of these experiences and put me on a new track of good experiences.* I didn't know how the development of the cure went. But if someone had gotten cured of the disease thanks to my donation, that seemed good enough. ...

I started blood donation 4-5 years ago when *I took charity works and donations seriously.* It all began when I was working at the South African Republic branch of Samsung. I had been working for Samsung for almost 17 years abroad, and it was my last overseas duty. In that country, I witnessed the extreme poverty among Africans. As a Christian, I started financing Christian missionaries in the country and accompanied them to mission sites at least once a year. ... I knew that there might've been people who made a greater success out of life than me. But I also knew that *I had a relatively successful life by luck. All by luck. I was thankful for that.* I was going to church, and I read about faith in the Bible. *My thankfulness was founded on religious faith.*

(Woo)

Goodwill Repayment for Enmity ("Paying Good for Evil")

Meanwhile, donors make goodwill repayments via plasma donation not only in return for preceding goodwill help and kindness. Some practice goodwill donations *in spite of* (Sung, Song, Han, and Gan) or *in response to* (Sun, Chang, and Dong) the social enmity and criticism that they have received since their infection. On the former occasion, what ultimately drives them to donate is the caring social relations that these potential donors realize and cherish all the more amid a surge of offensive criticisms of their infection. Surrounded by critical reactions from others, those who recovered from infection consider plasma donations as a way to appreciate and further consolidate these caring relations in their communities, like coworkers (Sung), friends (Han and Gan), and family (Song). This solidarity sometimes lies with unexpected, unknown social relations like fellow donors (Song). Solidarity among existing or novel social relations seems to give donors a renewed sense of belonging and existence. On the latter occasion, by contrast, donations are in direct response to critical reactions and social enmity. Driven by a strong moral decree like religious teaching (e.g., "love your neighbors" and "love your enemies"), people donate to reciprocate evil with good or to pay good for evil, with the hope to ultimately overwrite enmity – that they never aim for and yet has befallen them – with goodwill that they hope to carry on.

In either case, this initial cause of goodwill repayment for enmity tends to remain a relatively static, dominant cause throughout donations among donors (Sung, Han, and Song). That is probably because donations have been besieged from the beginning by a clear context of enmity toward the infected in the wider societal background. This relatively static way of signification contrasts with the dynamic evolution of the initial cause of goodwill repayment for goodwill help.

At the same time, the goodwill repayment for enmity is often made in terms of community-building among close others and fellow donors (Gan, Sun, Chang, and Dong). To the extent that the repayment donation is made regarding these multiple others who signify different meanings to donors, the initial cause evolves into comparably multiple meanings, such as community-building inside and outside the donors, confidence-building, new self-making, and cure-making.

There were two causes. Firstly, the hospital was doing many medical tests on me when I donated plasma. I thought these tests would be clearly helpful to me. Secondly, I was a public worker (a teacher), and many people were nervous about Covid-19. And there were quite some demands for antibodies. I saw the news that hospitals needed antibodies. As a public worker, I wanted to help. So, it was both for monitoring my health and helping others in need. …

The idea of plasma donation didn't get into me immediately after hospital discharge, though, *because I was stressed out as others blamed me a lot for the infection, and they showed no regard for my privacy.* It was one month after I was discharged from the hospital that I felt I was recovering from my fear of interactions with others and students. Fellow teachers at my school and my homeroom students were especially supportive, throwing a welcome party. These colleagues welcomed me back to school with all their hearts, although they had had to suffer at work and in quarantine due to my reckless infection.

Luckily, I was blessed with good people around me (i.e., 'inbok'). Thanks to them, *I was regaining composure, and the plasma donation news sank into my mind to pay them back. ... People who knew me didn't blame me but sympathized with me and encouraged me,* whereas *those unknown and anonymous on the internet were busy harassing me. Strangely, I suffered from the harassment and got depressed.* I could understand why some celebrities had killed themselves in response to what others said thoughtlessly.

Those close people, teachers, and students, however, stood beside me and pulled me out of depression and darkness. I wanted to thank them by repaying as much as I received. *My donation was meant for them. It wasn't any defiance against those who harassed me or the government that disappointingly mishandled my private information. I wasn't such a heroic kind of person (who defied adversaries) but an ordinary person. I looked at those who supported me despite it all. ... The donation didn't help me much to resolve the bad feelings that I got from those who hated me. ...* I was proud of myself for having donated when fellow teachers joked about me being the first antibody-carrier and the only one carefree with Covid-19 being around us. I did something that others couldn't even if they wanted to. They wanted to but couldn't help others, whereas I could help. *I realized that I was somebody that others needed. ...* I wanted to donate one more time at the same hospital. But it didn't take it anymore, and I didn't go to another donation center.

(Sung)

My year was full of bad luck, including the infection. ... *I was thinking I must do good things, like charity work, to end the string of bad luck I was having.* Then, I saw the donation ad. ... I wanted to help others in the ad, like those medical professionals. At the same time, *I wanted to make a break in the string of bad events in my life. I thought donation could be a moment for change. ...*

I talked to (three other) friends about it who had been infected together with me. *We had been together throughout the infection and in front of criticism from others.* Their first reaction was cynical, though. But *we talked about it again and decided to donate together. We* needed one good thing to stop bad things from happening. ... *Although we had been criticized a lot by others (for our infections), that didn't end up discouraging our donations.* Despite these people, we couldn't deny that there were medical professionals and the government that had helped us. They were *different people. ...*

It was my first plasma donation. It felt strange to see the fluid from my body that looked like pear juice. I wasn't fully persuaded that the liquid could help us. Anyway, I donated only because they said it would help. But *I wasn't sure. ...* I felt a little relieved by the news that

I had antibodies. … After all, I realized that I had done something good. I felt good about it and about myself.

(Han)

My friends and I talked about the donation ad. (We had worked for the same company for 6-7 years.) We went to the hospital *together* to get tested and see if we could donate. *We got together and decided to donate* it out of thankfulness to medical professionals. *We did it together.* I don't remember who suggested the idea first. It seemed that Gan and I tossed the donation news back and forth. *At some point, we (four friends) all agreed.* It's hard to tell who led us all. …

But I was a little hesitant at first. The hospital was too far, more than an hour away from my workplace. It was operating only during working days. Then, I saw news about good-willed donors like a married couple who had donated together in the hope of eradicating Covid-19 quickly. The news encouraged my friends and me. We concluded that *our donations might be helpful*, indeed. *We went there for donations two by two. Two friends donated together first. The other friend and I donated on another day, sitting next to each other* in the hospital for quite a while. … I went for donation light-heartedly, *as if I had gone for a drive. My friend was sitting next to me in my car.* There was nothing nervous or burdensome. I was filled with joy. …

Looking at the plasma coming out of my body, I didn't have any special feeling but simple curiosity. The staff said that they would run some tests on it. But *I didn't pay attention to what they exactly said about its uses.* … I was a little *relieved* after learning about my antibodies through the donation. …

I felt less guilty toward others after the donation. *It got rid of some of my guilt sense.* I became able to talk to others about my infection more openly. … Donation made me *feel that I did something,* although I didn't know what it was exactly. … *I knew that there were those who were blaming us for the infection, and there were others who had taken care of us and whom I would like to recognize.* … I would be able to donate again if I am asked to. *I am hooked up with these people (friends), after all.* … *After all that, we became even closer to one another.* It's like *the bonding feeling* among people who fought together at a battle.

(Gan)

I donated twice, traveling a long distance from Iksan to Seoul. It was *mostly due to my parents, who had insisted* that I should pay back this country that took care of me for free. They told me to act and volunteer for plasma donation. I agreed. That was how I made the first donation. … Although I had taken many drugs and injections at the treatment center, there had been no cure or enough information. *I wanted my donation to contribute to developing vaccines and drugs. I had that wish.* ... The government had spent a lot of money on my medical bill, which was around forty million wons (forty thousand US dollars). ... Then, one or two months later, I got a call from the hospital asking for another donation as I was being told about rich antibodies in me. I donated a second time. ...

I might've done it without my parents' suggestion. I would've done it to get rid of Covid-19 so that I could get my life back as well as all others'. ... *My parents had suffered a lot from others' hostile reaction* to my infection news. *But I took it not very seriously. Those hostile messages were anonymous anyway, and these people didn't know me, either.* I joked to my friends that they should respect me because *I sacrificed my blood for the common good and a better future, although others had oppressed my parents and me upon my infection.* ...

Blood-drawing was not different from common blood donation. What was different was *the sense of belonging in the donation room and the waiting room.* There were *other donors* who had all been infected in the past, and we had the experience in common and *talked about it lively*, like where each had been hospitalized, how long, and with what symptoms. It was so fun that it felt like seconds. We freely talked *with the hospital staff and the professor* with fun and smiles. It was like a cafe but coffee. ...

Once I learned about antibodies in me, I felt a little relieved. While most people were reeling back from public places in fear of infection, I acted like an exception and visited them carefree. ... When the hospital texted me that the patient got better thanks to my donated plasma, I felt proud that *I had done something for the patient.* I'd be willing to donate to a critically ill person one more time. ... If the first one was out of *obligation* for developing vaccines and cures, the second was with the sense of *sacrifice* for saving someone's life.

(Song)

The leader of the young adult group in the church posted a press release about the shortage in plasma donations nationwide to the online group chat room. It seemed that the members were thankful for the care they had received from hospitals and *wanted to pay back one way or another.* We talked to the pastor and leaders in the church about our willingness to donate. Then, the pastor talked to the city government, and they decided together to hold the official ceremony for *collective donation pledges. So, the initially small idea rolled into a rather official event.* There had been no clear procedure for taking donations in Busan. So, the city government stepped in to help our donations. ...

At that time, we had just started plans *to heal the outside of the church, or those in the local community whom the church congregation had hurt unintentionally with viruses.* Although the congregation itself had been a victim to Covid-19, we acknowledged that we had also threatened the local community with infection fear. So, the church started to hand out *goodwill gifts for the enmity that non-believers might've had toward us believers*. We wanted *to reciprocate any of our guilt with something good and benevolent*, like plasma donations and thank-you goodie boxes. *We wanted to revive ourselves and the local community at once out of the worries of Covid-19. That's what the church had been meant to be in the first place. We had wanted to share our love for the neighbors for a long time*. Although *Covid-19 had frustrated that wish and prayer with the unprecedented blame from the local community*, congregates put together their goodwill donations of plasma and distributed goodie boxes to neighbors. Congregates who hadn't been infected made whole blood donations for the same cause. ... My (Chang's) plasma donation was part of that effort. Although it wasn't very natural for me to step up, I submitted myself to the cause. ...

I (Sun) was representing the plasma donors. ... I was surprised at the number of reporters who showed up to cover *the donation pledges between our church and the city of Busan*. It was about 21 pledges in total. ... I would've hidden away and lived unnoticed if I hadn't stood up there in front of the press as the representative. I was hoping other members in the congregation would be encouraged by me and step up for donation. *We gathered up all the courage we had and managed to stand before the press.* ... We kept going. We believed that *collective donations* could help and suggested that *congregation members show their faces together to the public.* ... I (Sun) volunteered to be the donors' representative because I didn't want to let somebody who might've had some traumas risk being exposed to *external criticism toward the church* again. I was relatively free of trauma. I also had some free time to face potential threats on my terms. There were people among us who couldn't go to restaurants, meet people, or breathe well with others. ...

Our church and the city government originally planned to donate (transfuse) plasma directly to critically ill patients in the local hospitals. But the plan didn't go well. Instead, after several months, street donation centers opened in Busan. Each of the donors went to one of these centers and donated individually, although they had planned for collective donations. ... We saw that *people started having different attitudes toward our church after they knew of our donations, which helped some of us to get out of trauma*. People who had posted malicious comments about us online started posting *praises about us.* ... After co-workers knew about my (Sun's) donation, they called me an anti-body-carrier. They joked that I would certainly give them antibodies if they got infected by being around me. *It helped me to get back to social relations.* ... It was heart-warming. I (Chang) felt like I did something good and did a kind of charity work for others *as a member of society.* I wanted to do it one more time because the first donation *made me wish* for a quick end to Covid.

(Sun & Chang)

I posted news links about plasma donation to the group chat room among the congregation members who had been infected together. *Our church was suffering from a bad reputation from outside the community* just because the congregation members had been infected together on a big scale. People had been criticizing us believers for gathering for worship. It hurt me. *It was painful that non-believers were building up misunderstandings and negative impressions of the church.* I posted the news links, and the members all agreed on the idea. Pastors took our willingness forward. *We hoped that our donations might deliver our true intentions – neighborly love.*

(Dong)

Noblesse Oblige

The last cluster of donors starts drawing their plasma for the cause of social obligation. These donors state in common that the sense of duty and obligation toward the wider society and generalized others has been built in them as their nature at some points in life. Therefore, it feels like a self-sufficient, axiomatic deed to make convalescent plasma donations for a country that is in trouble collectively. This deed does not seem to be dependent on whether the donors feel and express gratitude for the country's support and help for the infection treatment (Seul, Ree, and Cheol) or whether they are put under undue social-relational hostility from others that can discourage any donations for the generalized others (Cheol). In this sense, these donations are unconditional and context-free. Some remote preconditions seem to be prior experiences of repeated donations of whole blood and college studenthood with time to look around (Seul), the unarticulated upbringing in the past that seemed to nurture the sense of responsibility (Ree), and the prestigious social statuses in education and vocation (Cheol).

In addition, this initial cause of noblesse oblige spawns emergent meanings of plasma donation, seemingly depending on how emphatically and concretely the donors refer to the cause. The more self-consciously the donors recall the cause of noblesse oblige (Cheol, compared to Seul and Ree), the more likely they ascribe additional meanings to their donations. Cheol embraces an array of emergent meanings, such as community-building (with his family as well as other potential donors), cure-making, science-making, confidence-building, and new self-making. Seul and Ree recall a smaller set of emergent meanings, such as confidence-building and new self-making (Seul) and immediate life-saving and new self-making (Ree).

I saw the news about plasma donation for cure development. *I immediately thought I could do it* because I had made standard (whole) blood donations many times. Plasma donation felt *like the standard blood donation*. At the same time, plasma donations could be made only by some but not all volunteers. This gave me *a stronger sense of duty and responsibility*. … As someone who had recovered from Covid-19, it seemed to be *something I should naturally do, like the standard blood donations* I was accustomed to. I had done it – standard whole blood donation – more than ten times then. *No matter what I had experienced at the moment of infection and in quarantine, those experiences didn't affect my decision whether to donate. Plasma donation was something natural and axiomatic* for me once I recovered. In addition, I was *a college student* with some free time. … At some point in my life, *I had accepted the idea of 'living together,'* which I had thought was only old men's saying. …

As for other causes, people were blaming those patients who got infected overseas, like me, for bringing back home the viruses and financial burdens. I didn't want to be unnecessarily a target of such criticism, although the social stigma surrounding me seemed never comparable to the enormous stigma that befell those who had been infected domestically and infected others around them as well. Anyway, it would've been good for all if anything (cure) had come out of my donation. I think *it was my nature and how I was built to have more social responsibility* than others. As soon as I saw the ad, I did it because I could. *I didn't think much about what my plasma would be used for.* I just thought it was for the public good. … The actual process was *so simple* that I sat there for one hour with needles in my arm, and it was done. I would've done it again if asked to. *It was nothing special.* … *While donating, I learned about antibodies formed in me, which relieved me a lot* because I was planning to go back to the UK to finish my study abroad. I thought antibodies would protect me abroad. … After the donation, I felt like *I became somebody a little special. I knew I did something, at least.*

(Seul)

As soon as I saw the TV ad, *I immediately called in.* It was only one or two days after the ad was aired. Initially, I thought it was for developing cures, but the KU Hospital called me to ask for a transfusion for an urgent patient once the hospital went through the basic tests on my body for a donation. It was rewarding to hear about the old patient in the 90s who got better after the transfusion. … *I don't remember any specific motivations in the beginning. Was there anything? I think I had been waiting for such an ad* because I knew about plasma donations in other countries. I was wondering why not in Korea. So, *I was already ready for it before it was publicized.*

Well, there were many reasons for me, maybe. I thought it (and a future cure from it) could be helpful to my family members, who might be infected later. I wanted to, I'm afraid it sounds bragging, be helpful to this country because it had taken good care of me for 45 days in the hospital. *Because I experienced how the UK government had treated its people in danger of Covid-19, I was very proud of this country.* It was the first time in my life taking such *pride in this country.* I thought it'd be very possible to develop cures and finish Covid-19 soon in this country. ... *I guess my personality was built that way.* I remained interested in the national community and *hoped to contribute the slightest change to the wide world. That's how I was made, and that's my personal belief. I'm sorry it sounds presumptuous.* ...

After the donation, *I felt proud of myself.* I felt like talking about it to others around me, but I didn't. I felt great for several days all by myself.

(Ree)

I had two competing thoughts. I didn't want to donate in one corner of my mind because a donation would reveal to others that I had been sickened from Covid-19. On the other, I wanted to do something in return for this country's support for me and my family. The latter was much stronger. *It was a sense of duty. I thought that's what justice meant.* ... I called in myself. After several (call) transfers, I talked to the KU Hospital about my intention. I said that *the government had cared for and benefited me and my youngest son (and my wife) for one and a half months,* and *the son was about to be conscripted for military duty.* I wanted to *donate together with my wife and son* if we were all qualified. ... It was to pay back what I owed.

I also wanted to add to the country's effort *to find cures.* Then, I heard on TV that there were not many donors. So, *I wanted to put up my donation as a public demonstration so that it could instigate other unwilling people.* I thought we could hope for cures only when there were many donors. ... When I got infected, some blamed me for the infection. I was shocked. But *I was somehow able to divert the sense of being unduly penalized and didn't blame them back.* That's probably because I knew in retrospect that I had responded to Covid-19 wisely in the early moments when no official guidelines had been in place yet. *I took pride in it, and I took relief in it. So, I donated (instead of blaming them back.)* ...

It was such *pride and obligation* that was behind it. In my generation, *I was one of those select few* who got a higher education at college.

Although I wasn't among those who gave all their wealth back to society as gifts, I had always been conscious of *social obligations and duty in my place. Plasma donation was one of them.* Then, one day, the head doctor of the donation project at the hospital asked me to be featured in an interview with the Hankyoreh (authors' note: one of the four major national newspapers) to boost the donation drive. I was caught between two thoughts. *I was one of the founding grassroots stock-funders of the newspaper when it was founded three decades ago, hoping to support an enlightened, new national news outlet.* So, I loved the idea of the interview. But my wife wouldn't support me because she was paranoid about disclosing our infection stories *to the nation.* I resigned, eventually. Anyway, I donated my plasma, which I thought was enough to *set an example for my kids and grandchildren.* My first child is an alum of Korea University, like me. The second one is a doctor of traditional Korean medicine who practices in the US. *My family members have been blessed by this country.* Even if not, *it still remains doubtless for people of those (prestigious) social statuses to donate* to the country. …

   Through the donation, I found myself having greater expectations for our country regarding future vaccines and cures. I could renew patriotism for our country, having seen its systematic and smart responses to Covid-19. … Thanks to the donation, I learned from a renowned professor at the hospital about antibodies in my body and important tips about how to fare amid Covid-19. I don't think all people can have such an opportunity. *There were many unexpected rewards.* I got a lung test from the renowned professor, a blood test, and an olfactory examination from another professor-specialist, all for free. So, I could learn much about my bodily conditions after the infection. I was paid for the travel expenditure as well. The press should've focused on covering *those unexpected but delightful and practical rewards* that donors could get from the already rewarding donations. The press was only covering the sensational and grandiose stories of a young folk who talked about the scary side effects of Covid-19, which didn't seem true to me, and his seemingly overstated accounts of plasma donations. *I hadn't anticipated those* reciprocal benefits. So, I was thankful for them. … *It's a self-evident law that I must return to the surrounding others what I've got from around for free,* like my *antibodies naturally formed from the infection.* When I follow this, it gives me *pride and hope.*

(Cheol)

4 Life Reassembled

Donors have encountered multiple meanings and causes developing from plasma donation. The extent to which plasma donation is concretized into various meanings and causes varies from donation to donation, making it an instance of liminality – i.e., instant liminality – that defies ready typifications and categorizations about what it means. This chapter describes that these varying ways in which people experience the instant liminality of plasma donation have impacts on how they reassemble the original liminality of life amid coronavirus disease-2019 (COVID-19) uncertainties. The chances for donors to appreciate multiple and often divergent meanings of plasma donation are higher among those with several simultaneous initial causes and those prone to developing emergent meanings in addition to initial causes. The more multiple meanings donors ascribe to plasma donation in either way, the more likely they are to do well with the COVID-19 liminality.

Plasma donations affect people's efforts to reassemble their lives amid the pandemic in two fashions. First, as far as donors experience plasma donation as developing multiple and sometimes unpredicted meanings and, nonetheless, being concretely and substantively present, they tend to normalize the original liminality that is likewise laden with conflicting, unfathomable experiences amid COVID-19 as something yet existent and livable if unfamiliar at a first look. Second, while donors are experiencing multiple meanings and causes that are joined together in plasma donation, they often observe that uncertain personal meanings are accompanied by collective, supra-individual certainties. As much as people acknowledge that plasma donation is made of both certainty and uncertainty in this manner, they take life amid the original liminality as harboring not only uncertainty but also certainty. For example, as much as donors experience personal worries and discontent about plasma donations meeting social-relational recognition of their acts of donation, supportive national healthcare systems for donors, medical-scientific knowledge and expertise surrounding donations, and unyielding commitments among professionals and close others toward donations, they learn to countenance worries

DOI: 10.4324/9781003493723-5

and disorders during COVID-19 with anticipation for hopes, orders, and unwavering anchors.

Still Disorderly Life After Donations

It is no surprise that plasma donation that can concretize into various causes and meanings, from awakening to new and old selves at an individual level to relational solidarity and scientific knowledge advancement at a societal level, materializes into a limited set of meanings among some donors. Surprising are the consequences of the plasma donations that generate few meanings for donors. When this happens for whatever reasons – donor–staff interaction-deprived donations on the street centers, even if donations are repeated twice (Bae) or the misfortunate lone donation despite the initial pledges for collective group donations (Kwang) – plasma donations produce little influence on how donors reconstitute their lives amid the COVID-19 liminality. Donors report little change after the donations in their sense of being worried, isolated, outcast, and on edge. Bae talks about persistent anxiety and seclusion despite repeated donations through which he has experienced only one emergent meaning of plasma donations – immediate life-saving – other than the initial cause of goodwill repayment for goodwill help. Kwang reflects on a similar sense of worry and being on the margin and threshold, not belonging firmly to his church community or other collectivities in a broader context. Kwang's initial cause for the donation – goodwill repayment for goodwill help – has barely led to another emergent meaning – community-building with fellow believers – in the middle of a foiled attempt for collective donations.

> I used to be pretty outgoing and like to hang out with people. But (after the infection, recovery, and plasma donation), *I find myself still unwilling to go to places packed with people.* I wouldn't go there. When I ever need to meet friends, I meet them in quiet places. It just happened so. I wasn't like that before. I used to call friends out to busy streets and bars. … But now I sometimes manage not to meet friends when I don't feel comfortable with the surroundings. So, *I meet friends and others less frequently than before.* That's because those people are not like family. I know a lot about family, like where they have been. But I've realized that *I don't know much about those people, like where they have been and what they have done before they come to meet me.* Speaking of close friends, I check their Instagram and other SNSs and know who likes to frequent bars and fun places. Then *I cannot afford to meet those friends because I don't know what these guys have made of all these.* … My neighbors? It's the same. Just like my friends, it feels natural to me to keep a distance from my neighbors, like in the

elevators. I don't know what they do for a living. Some of them may have to meet many strangers for work who may have been infected. So, I hesitate to hang out with neighbors. I have friends who run their own shops and businesses, and it's getting more difficult for me to meet them as I did. ... *I am anxious about me being infected again. That anxiety seems to stay with me, distancing strangers.* ... After some time since the first outbreak of Covid-19, other people seem to be going back to the old days, and I don't see much difference. *It seems to be only me who has changed in the attitude.* ... *I still remain watchful.* ...

Yes, people ask me many questions about Covid. They do so when they are nervous about Covid-19. But *they don't ask whether or how much I was suffering.* To put it simply, *people don't care about my lived experience, like what I was feeling and experiencing when I was quarantined in the hospital. They are usually curious about what I think about Covid-19.* (Interviewer: What do you mean?) Put simply, *they seem to want to know not my memory of the vivid experience of pains in the hospital but an overall bird's-eye reflection on it. They want to hear about what I think it was at the point when it was over.* How should I put it? Most others know what I had been doing before I went abroad (where I got infected) and how much I suffered in the hospital when I came back. *So, they don't ask about it, like, 'Was it okay in the hospital?' 'Was it good in Turkey?'* So, it's all disappeared. *It is five months from January (when I went abroad) to May (when I returned, got quarantined, and was discharged). Friends and others don't ask about these five months either because it is not necessary and pointless to them or because they don't want to remind me of the painful experience. They ask only about Covid-19 and not me or my five months. These five months are gone and lost.* The communication is superficial and not deep. It seems considerate in one sense. But it's not that simple. *These five months are all my experience and what I lived. That's what experience means. I had never foreseen or wanted any of those moments that happened to me, but they are nonetheless what I lived. My friends seem to think it is a golden rule not to ask me about these experiences for my sake.* If anyone ever asks about it, it is with a ton of precaution. Because they know how I was racially discriminated there and all that, ... They bring it up only over a drink as if it's a trivial matter. They don't talk about it when sober. ...

Speaking of whether we can overcome this pandemic, I believe we could. It's not a hard-evidenced belief, but it is so much a wish that anyone would have as an individual living in the present. In addition, I've been through it personally and am in my 20s, and I haven't had severe health events. It would be best if we could all escape from it, given those adverse side effects people have been talking about. If not, though, Covid-19 doesn't seem to be something that should make us panic.

(Bae)

But it (trauma) resurfaced out of nowhere in front of many people at an on-campus academic conference. I thought that I had gotten comforted to some degree by the anonymous supportive messages appended to the news reports of my infection story. (I had happened to be interviewed by the press once, and people reacted with supportive messages, which helped me.) But once I was put into this direct, in-person, face-to-face interaction with others at the conference, being unpredictably forced by my advising professor, *I fell apart. ... I've become extremely watchful* after all this. *It's cruel, but each person has to watch one's own back. There's no one else to do it for me.* I've come to take it deep into my heart. Even if I watch out, I may get infected. When I don't watch out for it myself, I certainly get infected. *I now put it all into my hands to take care of my surroundings*, whereas I used to think things get taken care of even behind my back. Now, it should be I who is in charge. ... Before and after the infection and donation, there is no difference in my anxiety about Covid-19. I know *I got infected for no reason, and I recovered for no reason (without a real cure). I dare not say I know about Covid-19.* I can only talk humbly about what I went through. I cannot be presumptuous, although I believe we don't need to get overly freaked out. ...

Because of the increasing number of infection cases nationally, the church has been asking us to refrain from gathering. *It seems that fellow believers and the church leadership are willing to embrace, help, and take in those who were once infected and now recovered like me. But*, since people cannot actually meet, *I don't feel like I am being accepted by them yet. ... I want others to take me as the completely cured. ... There remains the Kakao group chat room among fellow believers* who were once infected. (We used to exchange chats not only to inform others in quarantine but to plan for plasma donations together, although the donations didn't go as planned.) *But it is not very active, but it serves as a simple token that we have been through it together. We exchanged New Year's wishes but no special reflections about what we had been through.* ... Speaking of the worship on New Year's Eve, the congregation reflected on the past bumpy year amid Covid-19. But *it was a taboo to muse over where it all had begun in the church community. It was still traumatic.*

(Kwang)

Ever Orderly Life

The limited ramifications on donors' lives of the plasma donations to which donors ascribe meanings less progressively are palpable in another way. The second group of these donors remains unvaryingly sure of a good and stable life amid COVID-19 before or after their donations, constituting the opposite case to the experience of those who constantly remain precarious regardless of the donations. These donors have all initiated donations for the cause of goodwill repayment for enmity. They have made donations despite the aggressive, offensive reactions from unknown others. As the accompanying donation-driving factors, they have referred to good old coworkers (Sung), old friends (Han), and close family members (Song) through thick and thin. In a sense, these factors are not only the drivers for donations despite social enmity but also what enables the donors to feel secure, safe, and unswayed throughout the COVID-19 turbulences. Compared to the narratives of "still disorderly life after donations," these donors seem better off. On a second look, however, the narratives of "ever orderly life" lack plasticity and susceptibility that can resonate with the long-intractable, fluctuating pandemic situation in Korea as of 2020 and 2021. Lacking reflexivity and adhering to some obstinate strongholds like close people, these narratives seem as precarious as the pandemic situation remains out of touch with these strongholds.

> There isn't much change in life. Plasma donation wasn't a pivotal event but something little that *an ordinary person could do for close others.* I have always had *good teamwork with coworkers* at school. I am so satisfied with it that I haven't wanted to transfer to another school, although teachers can request a transfer across different schools every few years. My current coworkers seem to have the same satisfaction, working together for many years without a transfer request. I feel lucky. Before I became a teacher, I worked at a research institute, where I struggled with work relations with colleagues. I quit it. *I am blessed with good workplace relationships now, which has also helped me recover from Covid-19.* ...
>
> Although I am an irresolute Catholic who has been cooled down for the past ten years, I think it was thanks to God's help that I infected nobody. If anybody had been infected, I might not have recovered well (psychologically). So, I think I am lucky. *My life has been full of good luck, like good people around me (i.e., 'inbok'),* although it's not easy to relate it with God these days. ... *Thanks to good, close people, I think I am doing alright now.* ... Even when infection cases are increasing nationwide, I meet friends who jokingly say they feel the safest standing next to me. ... Students and parents get readily uneasy about Covid-19 when it seems to pick up its infection rate, even though most of them test negative. Then, *I talk casually* to students, 'Don't worry too much. It doesn't catch you easily if you keep up with the precautionary preventive measures.' *I freely tell* them that they didn't get infected when I was infected. ... *I am relieved.* Although many are worried about re-infection and new variants, I take solace in the fact that I have been through it.
>
> (Sung)

I don't think donation has changed my life much. ... *It's worrisome that Covid-19 is very infectious. Other than this, I think it is weaker than influenza*. It may be like a cold that goes away after two weeks. *I don't think it's a serious disease*, although people say it varies case by case.

(Han)

I have no fear. I have become brave, whereas others are living under the burden of Covid-19. I've already had it critically. I believe I wouldn't get another fatal disease. *I feel like I have already paid for it in advance. ... My close people remain the same. None has become distant from me. ... I don't think Covid-19 is a scary disease. It's only super-infectious.* We don't die of it, except for people with existing health conditions. I think it's like a common cold to healthy people. *I tell people not to worry.*

(Song)

Life as a Paradox

As donors confront multiple, diverse, and even conflicting meanings of their donations, such as confidence-building and confidence-threatening at once and both altruism and selfishness at once (Hee), they tend to accept that life during the pandemic is full of ailing, getting well, and falling sick again and that bodily recovery is not free from trauma and readily followed by relentless worries about reinfection. Life itself is described as a paradox that holds similarly contradictory elements together, like the strong will for dominance over difficult feelings in the heart and, simultaneously, the ready acquiescence with those feelings, and both the surreptitious wish to get away from kids and the outright caring to love them back. This constitutes a third way to react to the COVID-19 liminality: to see life as inherently paradoxical as plasma donation is.

Going through infection and plasma donation, ... *I came to accept that I could live my life in a selfish way. ... It's an irony. I realized no event had simply one meaning. ... I am soft-voiced and shy. But I'm also bold and gutsy. ... The bottom line is nobody is perfect, like my apartment neighbors who criticized me for being infected and harmful to them but welcomed my story because it got their apartments nationwide attention and pushed up the market recognition.* We are all the same. I came to know that. At times, I simply wasn't able to accept those people because I wasn't in the mindset. When I find peace in my heart again, I will be able to smile and meet those people. *I accept it all.*

Bodily recovery, socializing, and then recurring trauma all seem to me to be what life is. While living, we simply have accidents and sufferings. *Life has it all. ... I wanted to confront my problems and my feelings face to face and overcome them. But I don't seem to triumph over what's in my heart*. I will only have to live with it. … *Whether I am ready or not, my little kids are clinging to my skirt, asking for things. Then, I have to love them back.*

(Hee)

Disorderly Life with an Outlook for Certainty

To donors who have suffered substantially from social-relational hostility due to infection, although encountering a moderate set of different emergent meanings of plasma donation in addition to the initial cause of confidence-building (Min) and those who have donated for the initial cause of noblesse oblige and have not experienced – but always expecting for unfulfilled – many additional emergent meanings (Seul), life amid COVID-19 is yet filled with uncertainties and worries. At the same time, to the extent to which they have witnessed, if moderately (Min) – and have hoped to witness, being driven unabatedly by the noblesse oblige norm (Seul) – plasma donations evolving into various causes and meanings, some of which are generative of positive outlooks for the future, if unpredicted at the moment of donations, they try to remain optimistic about how COVID-19 will end for their lives. These narratives are dominantly about ordeals and confusion amid COVID-19, yet are qualified by the hope for the better. Personal, momentary struggles do not necessarily preordain a societal meltdown forever (Seul).

> Once I have been through it all, *I am still more worried than relaxed about Covid-19.* It was a difficult time for me. I wish nobody around me needed to go through it. I would never suffer it again. Although the necessary quarantine period is shortened now, *the fact that one is easily at risk and a risk to others is quite unbearable, much more so than one can guess.* It's stressful, full of worries, and makes one think of many things. *So, I take every possible precaution not to be infected again.* I get gloomy when the number of national infection cases increases from time to time. … *But the public news media shouldn't be so sensational. They shouldn't describe it in such a nerve-racking manner.* Speaking of the side effects from the symptomatic treatment in quarantine, for example, I didn't have any. Neither did my brother. But, some news media reported that 90% of the infected underwent side effects, which isn't simply true. It gives the wrong impression that almost all the once infected are sick in one way or another, even after being released from quarantine. *Such an inflammatory approach doesn't help us at all. Help lies somewhere else.*

(Min)

Nothing has changed fundamentally. I was disheartened when my last years in college didn't go as I had planned, like one semester of study abroad and the subsequent two semesters for preparing for the job market. *But I am just taking it in now. … Covid-19 wouldn't get this whole society into trouble forever. But it is only that I struggle to rebalance my plans* after the infection as the available jobs are decreasing. *It is not certain* how things will go.

(Seul)

Orderly Life with a Few Loose Ends

For a majority of donors who have partaken of a dynamically evolving set of meanings while donating plasma, life with COVID-19 is represented as orderly with a few unwieldy loose ends. As these donors embrace and encounter multiple possibilities – foreseen and novel – regarding what plasma donation means for their post-infection struggles – more so than the previous four groups of donors – they tend to accept as complex aspects of livelihood during the pandemic. Given their endorsement of divergent elements in life at once, their attitude toward life seems ambivalent and vulnerable on the one hand; on the other, it is flexible and generative, being reflexive not only of the persistent threats of virus infections in the surroundings but also of many ways of countering these threats and, ultimately, forging opportune footholds for the better across both threats and countermeasures, such as striking out the middle ground instead of leaning to the extremes (Gan); circumspection (Wook); experiential knowledge and expertise (Cheol); belief in individuals' persevering capacity and future remedies (Jin); trust in medicine and God's care (Sun and Chang); collective suffering, condolence, sympathy, and encouragement (Dong); the compromised and yet confident living along with viruses (Hwan); renewed self-confidence and patriotism (Sook); and, finally, donations and charity work (Woo). Compared to the monotonous outlooks on livelihood during the pandemic – i.e., the narratives of a still disorderly life and an ever-orderly life – these variants of orderly life with loose ends are each multivocal and sophisticated. Whereas the view of life as a paradox is static and ambivalent, this view of life as being orderly with unwieldy parts is dynamic and multivalent.

There is no other way but to meet people with care. It's impossible never to meet others or to meet others without fear of infection. *It's all by luck.* I talk with others about Covid-19 *not very seriously or too lightly.* Although people are very serious about it, *I tell them it's not so threatening. … I worry about it. But I am not anxious.* Since I have been through it, I tell myself, *'I know you.'* So, I only watch out for it.

(Gan)

I've come to appreciate what I used to take for granted, like going to my favorite restaurants in the neighborhood whenever I wanted to. One day in May, breathing in the spring air was so great after I secretly pulled down the mask in an open space with nobody around. It sounds like no big deal, but there is an unmistakable change in how I take in daily routines that I used to presume. *I've come to treasure every moment of the daily routine I can live because there are so many routines I cannot enjoy anymore.* All along, *I've become more watchful about what I do and shouldn't do daily.* I am probably more compliant with the preventive measures against Covid-19 than other people. *I watch out* for strangers and those who do not wear masks and talk a lot. I try not to go to crowded places. I have realized that accidents happen momentarily. We all know that. As soon as I loosen up and go easy with rules, saying they are too much and it's gonna be okay without them, then accidents occur. ... *Ever since I learned about antibodies in me thanks to the donation, I've become relieved a little and believe I will be okay and I can survive. But, as I've been saying, I also think that infection will come back anytime when I am off guard.* It's like I am going through a cycle. *While I mostly loosen up, I readily curl up and become vigilant if things don't look easy.* I do this repeatedly.

(Wook)

Do people call it trauma? Yes, I have such a feeling. It's been over one year since the infection, but I still hesitate to talk to others about it. Today, I am talking about it with you. ... *I wouldn't say I am peaceful now. But I'm experienced.* Isn't it that scholars of future studies predict infectious diseases will still come one after another? So, I may be infected again at any time. But the bottom line is *I know what to do to viruses and people (and to my body). I've learned from my experience. I've got an edge* over others who haven't experienced it.

(Cheol)

It's been over one year since the Covid-19 outbreak. We still have many infection cases. People are filled with fears, although there are different levels among people. *I don't think we should stay scared. Yes, it is scary when it develops into critical cases.* ... But *I am optimistic about cures being developed. I look forward to it.* ... Nobody predicted Covid-19 coming. I didn't expect that I would get infected. As much as that's true, it is also true that I can be infected anytime if things go that way. So, yes, *I will be doing my best to comply with precautionary measures and prevent it from happening. But there are things beyond personal efforts and individual powers. I accept it.* ... *I am not nervous. I have been through it once, so I have become solid.* I know how it would go if I were infected again, although I wish not. Others seem to be scared more than necessary because they haven't experienced it. *Viruses are scary, though.*

(Jin)

We both believe that *we would be alright (under God's guidance)*. We have recovered, after all. Nevertheless, I (Sun) wouldn't go through it again. *I trust medicine.* But I personally cannot accept the situation where my life gets blocked again. ... I (Chang) don't get super-paranoid about Covid-19. I am not fearful. But I don't want to go through it one more time because *I know the suffering. There are uncertainties* about Covid-19. *But I seem to be less scared* of them compared to other people.

(Sun & Chang)

I don't see much change in my social relations and how I meet people because of Covid-19. By the way, I have a friend's wedding to attend in two weeks. When I think about it now (compared to weddings before Covid-19), *Covid-19 seems to be still damaging my life. That's how it is, although I haven't realized it until I think of the wedding.* ... There is no guarantee that I won't be infected again. *I always have that insecurity.* ... I seem to have *two different feelings about Covid-19.* ... It is an unknown disease without any cure yet. Anybody can be infected at any time. So, many people fear it. *Everything is up in the air. It is up to heaven.* I think we should stop fault-finding and finger-pointing. *Instead, we should sit next to someone who is infected, commiserate with the person, and encourage the person.* We need to tell the person that it's *not a personal fault* and we can overcome it together. *Condolence, sympathy, and encouragement* are the most important. I don't think we can eradicate Covid-19. *We may have to bear with it, live with it, and thus find ways to help one another.*

(Dong)

It seems impossible to recover fully from Covid-19. Hospital discharge is one thing, and full recovery is another. I have lost some hair due to the adverse effects of the treatment I got. I know others kept going to hospitals due to lingering respiratory symptoms. I heard of someone who went back to the ICU after hospital discharge. There are episodes of adverse effects like brain fog, skin color changes, and chronic fatigue. *Getting better sounds more appropriate than full recovery. ... There is no full recovery.* Even though people call us the cured who have recovered, they keep generating suspicion, doubts, and oppressive criticisms of us. Since this is the true reality, *I like to be called someone who is getting better rather than someone who has recovered.* ... I once wrote this, and I believe this is right. *It is more important to be ready to accept living with Covid-19 than to look forward to cures.*

I have heard from experts that it will take two to ten years to have cures available in the market. If that's true, *I think it's right to accept life with Covid-19 and to plan a happy life amid the constrained daily routines with Covid-19.* I believe we have to accept this incomplete, constrained life as reality instead of complaining about it. *We may have to give up some things that we did before Covid-19. Still, we can be happy, and we need to try to be happy.*

(Hwan)

I am carefree with Covid-19, about 80%, I'd say. I've almost forgotten that I was once infected. But, when my daughter was about to visit me from abroad, it came back into my mind. My infection experience came alive. So, *I'd say about 80% of daily routines are back. I don't think I'd get infected again.* Still, I am curious about what doctors and nurses say about my odds of being infected again. Do you think it's okay to stay with my daughter at home only if she tests negative (when she visits me next time)? ... *I am still in fear of Covid-19.* When I had a chest strain recently, I was deeply worried and went to the hospital for an MRI test. I was traumatized by pneumonia that I had had from Covid-19. The MRI result was good, though. Whenever I have a concern, I run to the hospital. But *I have more confidence and trust in myself now*, compared to the past. ... I used to think of myself as weak. *I now know I am a healthy kind of person.* And, although it's a big story, *I now see this country on the bright, positive side* if another crisis comes.

(Sook)

People have their own ways of confronting and getting out of trouble. I go to church. I turned and relied on religion and faith a lot. I frequently went to twilight worship because I had no work to do anyway. Then, I participated in plasma donation because I needed *one moment* to get out of the difficulties. I believed that even *a small service to others* would provide me with chances to feel thankful for my life being of any use to others, and *this gratitude would be part of the process of overcoming my difficulties.* I believed it would be *the moment* to overcome life crises. ... As a matter of fact, it did result in some ways to overcome the difficulties. Plasma donation brought gratitude to my mind; in turn, *thankfulness brought about good things around me, of course, along with bad things, though.* I had been fired by my lifelong employer, set up a business, and almost immediately closed it down, suppressed by Covid. I had wanted to put all these behind me, go forward, and be positive toward the future. *Plasma donation was there. There will be other crises in the future, and I believe I will be donating in goodwill and become able to overcome them.*

(Woo)

Conclusion

What do we learn from this book regarding liminality, gifts, donations, and sociology? *Liminality* is a sociological language that aims not to fail to describe and design human experiences that defy and extend beyond taken-for-granted categories, patterns, and structures. It is a promising language for not only studying but also experiencing the living facts that are not dead but real, yet elusive and challenging. It is the reality that people must live through when existing systems and knowledge are helpful yet insufficient, let alone when they are doubtful. By listening to the voices of people who have lived in such a reality during the pandemic, this study proposes an alternative theoretical model that renews the existing wisdom.

The literature has so far informed three pieces of wisdom separately. It reports when and how individuals turn liminal, what they do in response to liminality, and the different consequences of liminality for their lives. Although each makes its own contributions, it has accordingly remained unclear whether different ways of turning liminal and/or different ways of responding to liminality lead to different consequences. While some report destructive consequences of liminality and others report generative ones, not enough effort has been made to examine both possibilities simultaneously by heeding the accompanying contexts. To fill these gaps, this study puts together a full round of narratives from people in liminality and proposes a holistic theorization that connects these pieces.

By so doing, it provides a formal representation of how liminality remains central to human existence that classics have long suggested. This study formalizes human existence – i.e., a life process – as a unique dialectical process between original problematic liminality and ensuing instant liminality. First, since a life process refers to a series or combination of categories and non-categories, it readily exists in non-categories and, thus, manifests itself as problematic liminality, like infection during the pandemic. Second, individuals respond to problematic liminality with other practices that defy ready categorization and signification – i.e., instant liminality – like plasma donations. How instant liminality is concretized

DOI: 10.4324/9781003493723-6

into categories and meanings is partly conditioned by problematic liminality and partly contingent upon the opportune developments internal to instant liminality itself. Third, the ways in which instant liminality concretizes itself ultimately reshape original liminality. This study argues that original problematic liminality ends up being either only destructive or both destructive and generative, depending on how instant liminality unfolds. This argument complicates the existing literature that bifurcates the consequences of liminality into being either destructive or generative. Taken together, this study proposes that people live through liminality by relying not only on certainties and categories but also liminalities – all of which are conceptualized as variants of liminality in this study – with varying consequences. This life journey is worth naming *liminalization*.

The gift is another sociological language that heeds life's irreducible yet challenging plurality that defies and exists beyond rigid categorization, reduction, and concretization. Accounting for the necessary exchanges and gift-giving among individuals, Mauss has found oxymorons – like a free obligation and obliged freedom – and couplings – between material and immaterial interests or between physical and metaphysical forces in the world – to be essential to all gifts and social relations at large. While Mauss progressively reaches the structuralist-sounding notion of totality out of oxymoron, coupling, and multiplicity, later studies largely agree on multivocality and multivalence in gifts and donations in less structuralist and more phenomenological manners. In response to the literature, this study shows that totality is processually experienced as multivocality – or, processual multivocality hints at structural totality – and, more importantly, that multivocality – at times, appreciated as liminality – can be an effective way to live through liminality, to which the studies of the gift have paid little attention yet. Giving and donations are not made without effort on the side of donors. A donor makes gifts to become a total human being and service to others, to the maximum, or a multivocal being to the minimum. To the extent to which this effort is realized, gifts and donations varyingly reconstitute the donor's life in liminality and beyond. Likewise, beneficiaries do not receive gifts without effort. Depending on what effort they make and the extent to which their effort is materialized in actual gift relations, gifts may have varying impacts on reshaping receivers' lives that are partly known and partly unknown to the receivers.

Are liminality and the gift promising *sociological* languages beyond the pandemic context, adaptable to other lived experiences of individual existence and agency in the world? Regarding what social sciences in general and sociology in particular – vis-à-vis (natural) science – should be like, Parsons enthusiastically argues that social sciences should accept "the fact that man stands in significant relations to aspects of reality other than those revealed by science. Moreover, the fact that empirical reality can be modified by action shows that this empirical reality, the world of science, is not a closed system but is itself significantly related to the other aspects of reality" (Parsons, 1935, p. 290). He continues on the same page that "while our logical formulations of non-empirical reality differ from those of empirical reality – that is, are not scientific theories – they exist none the less. They are metaphysical theories, theologies, etc." In the end, to Parsons, "the real", the sociological reality, or human existence/agency is composed of the transcendental and metaphysical on the one hand and the empirical and positivist on the other.

This fundamental duality – and plurality, in a proper extension – of reality and human existence has been long recognized among classical sociologists. "We are constantly seeking ultimate forces, fundamental aspirations, some one of which controls our entire conduct. But in no case do we find any single force attaining a perfectly independent expression, and we are thus obliged to separate a majority of the factors and determine the relative extent to which each shall have representation. (...) An action that results from less than a majority of fundamental forces would appear barren and empty. (...) Human life cannot hope to develop a wealth of inexhaustible possibilities until we come to recognize in every moment and content of existence a pair of forces, each one of which, in striving to go beyond the initial point, has resolved the infinity of the other by mutual impingement into mere tension and desire" (Simmel, 1957 [1904], p. 541). Thus, Simmel proclaims, "man has ever had a dualistic nature".

Once having famously typified action into being instrumental-rational, value-rational, affectual, and traditional, Weber states that "it would be very unusual to find concrete cases of action, especially of social action, which were oriented only in one or another of these ways. Furthermore, this classification of the modes of orientation of action is in no sense meant to exhaust the possibilities of the field, but only to formulate in conceptually pure form certain sociologically important types to which actual action is more or less closely approximated or, in much the more common case, which constitute its elements" (Weber, 1978 [1922], p. 26). Therefore, rationalization, which means the dynamic process of a subject's mastering over life matters in the world, refers to contingent alignments – or, elective affinities – among various kinds of rationality and action logic that are already known – like those represented as the value spheres of life – and yet to be known (Howe, 1978; Kalberg, 1980; McKinnon, 2010).

In these exemplary quotes, the essential sociological task lies in illuminating – and providing people with tools to appreciate – how the fundamental flow of life process is concretized with some patterns and categories, without leading the attention to the latter to neglecting the former and vice versa, and without reducing the former to the latter nor assuming the former without the latter. Berger and Luckmann (1991 [1967]) formalize this task as the sociology of knowledge, which is concerned first and foremost with ordinary people who lead their daily lives being both sure and doubtful that they know the reality – i.e., everyday life with both knowledge and ignorance at once, with knowns and unknowns simultaneously, and with one kind of knowledge along with another. In their own terms, "the man in the street inhabits a world that is 'real' to him, albeit in different degrees, and he 'knows,' with different degrees of confidence, that this world possesses such and such characteristics" (Berger & Luckmann, 1991 [1967], p. 13). The man in the street lives and exists in knowledge – the subjective, inclusive of one's own body, soul, and mind, we interpret – and reality – the objective, involving others' body, soul, and mind. Sometimes, the two overlap, while they diverge other times. This whole process of knowledge and reality, or the everyday life of a man in the street living in multiplicity and tensions of knowledge and reality, is what the social construction of reality means in the book – i.e., reality that is a construct of many things.

The tensions of knowledge and reality are nothing more than those of one knowledge with another, which opens the door to the infamous relativism regarding knowledge. One person's knowledge is different from another's. A person's current knowledge is relative to the person's future knowledge. One culture or wisdom is relative to another civilization or sapience. Many would habitually accept that relativism is no good for science. Although tempted to agree so easily, one must contemplate what relativism fundamentally means in Berger and Luckmann before yielding to the attraction. What is ultimately relative and thus unstable is knowledge *in relation to* reality. Any knowledge and knowing are relative to reality, so knowledge diversifies into different kinds – each of which has its own relation to reality – and produces schisms and tensions. Therefore, one firm way to get rid of relativism in knowledge is to disconnect controllable, visible knowledge from intractable, invisible reality and let only the visible agree with one another. One would get absolute knowledge for its own sake but at the cost of losing interest in living in reality with the help of knowledge. An alternative to getting stable, absolute knowledge is to hold the reality still that knowledge relates to. Then, one would get knowledge that interests the person in a reality that is stable and certain. One could sustain interest in living in reality with such knowledge. However, what kind of reality is this? It is a reality that is still, dormant, and unchanging. If that is the reality that one lives in, one can hardly say that one is *living*. Living is a process but not a permanent state.

In all, knowledge relativism means nothing but reality relativism, which means instability, wildness, wilderness, unfathomability, and "darkness" (Berger & Luckmann, 1991 [1967], p. 59) in reality, which, in turn, guarantees the real-ness of living. For the very sake of living, knowledge relativism and reality relativism are crucial and absolute. If one may call it infamous, relativism is the absolute, inalienable foundation of life, which is "dark", "taken for granted", "already unproblematic", and "things that go on 'behind my back'" (Berger & Luckmann, 1991 [1967], pp. 38, 59). What is genuinely *problematic* for individuals is to embrace this absolute yet challenging relativism – plurality, in other words – by being able to taste, experience, express, and illuminate their living in the darkness with the help of objects, types, and institutions. Berger and Luckmann call this life process objectivation/objectification, typification, and institutionalization.

This book suggests liminalization and gift-making in their places. It shows that *liminalization* – simply put, living through original problematic liminality with instant liminality, or processing the underlying fundamental liminality with many instant liminalities – and *gift-making* – i.e., wrapping heterogeneities in a rewarding whole, like in a gift box – are some of such social practices. To the extent that individuals exist forcibly or willingly outside firm categories, and as long as people exchange various immaterial, vague aspirations with material, concrete goods, these languages will suffice for the fundamental sociological work and social practice beyond the pandemic. At one of those junctions, this book concludes that, when facing the great unknown now and then, people curl up on a concrete act that not only delivers finite meanings but is also generative of unknown, unpredicted meanings that unfold only in the act and thus shed light on the great unknown.

References

Berger, P. L., & Luckmann, T. (1991 [1967]). *The social construction of reality: A treatise in the sociology of knowledge.* Penguin Books.

Howe, R. H. (1978). Max Weber's elective affinities: Sociology within the bounds of pure reason. *American Journal of Sociology, 84*(2), 366–385. https://doi.org/10.1086/226788

Kalberg, S. (1980). Max Weber's types of rationality: Cornerstones for the analysis of rationalization processes in history. *American Journal of Sociology, 85*(5), 1145–1179. http://www.jstor.org/stable/2778894

McKinnon, A. M. (2010). Elective affinities of the protestant ethic: Weber and the chemistry of capitalism. *Sociological Theory, 28*(1), 108–126. http://www.jstor.org/stable/25746216

Parsons, T. (1935). The place of ultimate values in sociological theory. *International Journal of Ethics, 45*(3), 282–316. http://www.jstor.org/stable/2378271

Simmel, G. (1957 [1904]). Fashion. *American Journal of Sociology, 62*(6), 541–558. https://doi.org/10.1086/222102

Weber, M. (1978 [1922]). *Economy and society: An outline of interpretative sociology* (Vol. 1, G. Roth & C. Wittich, Eds.). University of California Press.

Index

For Product Safety Concerns and Information please contact our EU
representative GPSR@taylorandfrancis.com
Taylor & Francis Verlag GmbH, Kaufingerstraße 24, 80331 München, Germany

www.ingramcontent.com/pod-product-compliance
Ingram Content Group UK Ltd.
Pitfield, Milton Keynes, MK11 3LW, UK
UKHW021123180425
457613UK00006B/203